BORN TO DIE

NEW APPROACHES TO THE AMERICAS

edited by Stuart Schwartz, *Yale University*

BORN TO DIE

DISEASE AND NEW WORLD CONQUEST, 1492–1650

NOBLE DAVID COOK

Florida International University

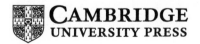
CAMBRIDGE
UNIVERSITY PRESS

PUBLISHED BY THE PRESS SYNDICATE OF THE UNIVERSITY OF CAMBRIDGE
The Pitt Building, Trumpington Street, Cambridge CB2 1RP, United Kingdom

CAMBRIDGE UNIVERSITY PRESS
The Edinburgh Building, Cambridge CB2 2RU, United Kingdom
40 West 20th Street, New York, NY 10011-4211, USA
10 Stamford Road, Oakleigh, Melbourne 3166, Australia

First published 1998

Printed in the United States of America

Typeset in Goudy Old Style 10½/13

Library of Congress Cataloging-in-Publication Data

Cook, Noble David.
Born to die : disease and New World conquest (1492–1650) / Noble
David Cook.
p.   cm. – (New approaches to the Americas)
Includes bibliographical references and index.
ISBN 0-521-62208-5 (hc.) – ISBN 0-521-62730-3 (pbk.)
1. Indians – Diseases.   2. Epidemics – America.   3. Indians –
Population.   4. America – History – To 1810.   I. Title.   II. Series.
E59.D58C66   1998
614.4'97 – dc21   97-25064

A catalog record for this book is available from the British Library.

ISBN 0-521-62208-5 hardback
ISBN 0-521-62730-3 paperback

040898-483602

To
Cuitláhuac and Huayna Capac
and the millions
who fell not to the sword
but to the
unseen foe within

Great was the stench of the dead. After our fathers and grandfathers succumbed, half of the people fled to the fields. The dogs and the vultures devoured the bodies. The mortality was terrible. Your grandfather died, and with them died the son of the king and his brothers and kinsmen. So it was that we became orphans, oh my sons! So we became when we were young. All of us were thus. We were born to die!

Annals of the Cakchiquels, ca. 1559–81

Contents

Tables, Illustrations, and Maps

Tables

Illustrations

Maps

ACKNOWLEDGMENTS

The excitement of historical research and discovery creates a bond linking an international scholarly community. My initial investigations into the relation of epidemic disease to the demographic collapse of Amerindian America began many years ago, as I searched for the causes of the total disappearance of some groups while others survived. Dobyns's conference "Native American Historic Demography," held at the Newberry Library in Chicago in December 1983, forced me to rethink my arguments on the role of disease in the conquest of the Americas. At that time we were working independently on developing epidemic disease models to estimate aboriginal population size. Dobyns's enthusiastic encouragement was and is always appreciated. At the Newberry conference I first met historical geographer W. George Lovell. A common intellectual curiosity centering on the European's impact on Amerindian people – his on the Quiche Maya of Guatemala, mine on the Quechua and Aymara of highland South America – soon led to an enriching academic relationship. In 1986 we participated in a symposium on colonial migrations organized by David J. Robinson at Syracuse University, where, during evenings of stimulating and often heated discussions with specialists Elsa Malvido, David Robinson, John Kicza, and Robert McCaa, Lovell and I decided to chair jointly a symposium on disease in Hispanic America for the 46th International Congress of Americanists, scheduled to meet in Amsterdam in July 1988. There, presentations by regional specialists representing several disciplines provided the foundation for an edited volume, *Secret Judgments of God*, confined chronologically and spatially to colonial Spanish America. Yet epidemics cannot be geographically restricted to one part of the New World, for at the time movement through normal exchange networks between ethnic entities was continuous. Furthermore, even after the arrival of the Europeans, quarantine was imperfect and remedies for disease were ineffective. The seeds of several of the chapters of the present work were planted at regional and international conferences. Martin S. Kenzer's invitation to participate in the 19 March 1989 Annual Meeting of the American Geographical Society in Baltimore, Maryland, and to review William M. Denevan's paper "Carl Sauer and Native American Population Size in the New World" compelled me to focus attention on the subject of Hispaniola's pre-contact numbers and on the reasons for the virtual disappearance of the island Taino. Research for the abbreviated comments on Denevan's paper finally evolved into Chapter 1. An incomplete early version was published in *Colonial Latin American Review* 2(1993):213–45. Many of the themes developed in Chapter 2 took form during investigations for participation in Verena Stolcke and Juan Martínez-Alier's Spring 1990 conference "New Anthropological, Demographic and Ecological Perspectives of the Conquest of America" held at the Universitat Autónoma de Barcelona. A small part of Chapter 3 stems from research for a paper on epidemics in the Andean area prepared for a November 1989 Smithsonian Institution conference on "Disease and Demography in the Americas" that was chaired by Douglas H. Ubelaker and John W. Verano. The remainder of the text is fresh.

I thank especially the John Simon Guggenheim Memorial Foundation, which provided a generous fellowship for the academic year 1991–92 that allowed me precious time to proceed on the project. I also appreciate the support of Frederick Holmes, Chair of the History of Medicine Division of the Yale University Medical School, who graciously facilitated my appointment to that institution as research affiliate, and in so doing provided me with full access to its remarkable research collections. The staff of the Libraries of Yale University assisted as attentively in this project as in prior investigations. In a similar vein, the Interlibrary Loan Department of Florida International University worked overtime to secure vital published texts.

As always, my principal mentor and companion is Alexandra Parma Cook; she is also my best and most enthusiastic critic, a rare combination. She provides a realistic perspective when administrative and teaching responsibilities compete for time. Furthermore, she has always been ready to sacrifice her own schedule to comment on and help to polish paragraphs, pages, and chapters as the manuscript moved forward. Her own sweeping history has been too long delayed. My debt is great, as are my respect and affection. That debt will be repaid. Karoline Parma Cook's keen eye is also appreciated. Anonymous readers provided insightful commentary. Kenneth F. Kiple shared timely counsel on potential sources for funding at an important juncture in my research and writing, and with the completion of the text, he read and made critical suggestions for improvements. His comments on yellow fever and malaria have led me to rethink some conclusions on these maladies. Nicolás Sánchez-Albornoz, who directed early steps in the field of historical demography, continues to inspire by example. Of course, errors in fact and interpretation are solely my own.

Born to Die

The biological mingling of the previously separated Old and New Worlds began with the first voyage of Columbus. The exchange was a mixed blessing: It led to the disappearance of entire peoples in the Americas, but it also resulted in the rapid expansion and consequent economic and military hegemony of Europeans. Amerindians had never before experienced the deadly Eurasian sicknesses brought by the foreigners in wave after wave: smallpox, measles, typhus, plague, influenza, malaria, yellow fever. These diseases conquered the Americas before the sword could be unsheathed. From 1492 to 1650, from Hudson Bay in the north to southernmost Tierra del Fuego, disease weakened Amerindian resistance to outside domination. The Black Legend, which attempts to place all of the blame for the injustices of conquest on the Spanish, must be revised in light of the evidence that all Old World peoples carried, literally though largely unwittingly, the germs of the destruction of American civilization.

INTRODUCTION

From the time of the great explorers of the Age of Reconnaissance, people have wondered how a mere few hundred Spaniards, with a small number of allies, were able to conquer two of the largest empires known at the time: the Aztec and the Inca. Why did some survive, whereas others succumbed so precipitously to the outsiders who reached the shores of the West Indies at the end of the fifteenth century? How were seemingly densely inhabited islands denuded of their aboriginal residents so quickly, to be replaced by foreigners who, after their own deadly seasoning period, multiplied marvelously? It seemed that everywhere in the New World, within three or four generations, a brief yet tragic period, strangers became the dominant force, ruling over an increasingly meager and weak native populace.

In the sixteenth century, two principal explanations were offered. One, best portrayed by the arguments of the "Protector of the Indians" Friar Bartolomé de Las Casas (1474–1566), stressed the cruelty of the Spaniards as the main factor that led to European dominance and native subjugation. The Iberians killed, maimed, and in every way possible made miserable the Indians they enslaved. This so-called Black Legend of Spanish evil was a powerful explanation, one that other European nations seized on with relish, for it justified their own encroachments on the territories and peoples of an alien and "evil" Catholic empire. The counterexplanation for the demise of the Amerindian peoples was religious. Christian friars and theologians could not fathom the reason the Indians, once so prevalent, seemed to be doomed to extinction. The cause must be providential, in one way or another associated with God's secret plan to foster the quicker spread of the Faith to all people or to punish the natives for presumed crimes

1

against nature – cannibalism, human sacrifice, sodomy, even their
frequent and unexplained rejection of the Word. Bartolomé de Las
Casas, in diverse texts, provides a host of examples of the most horren-
dous acts of sadism imaginable. Cruelty was not limited to excesses
committed against enemy warriors in the heat of battle; it extended to
the young and innocent. For example, a pair of Spaniards, so-called
Christians,

> met two twelve-year-old Indian boys one day, each carrying a
> parrot; they took the two and just for pleasure beheaded the
> boys. Another tyrant, angry at an Indian chief because he did
> not do what he ordered, hanged twelve of his vassals, and an-
> other one eighteen, all in one house. Another one shot arrows
> into an Indian following a public announcement that he was
> sentencing him because he was not quick enough in bringing
> him a letter that was sent to him. There are infinite cases and
> deeds of this nature that our Christians have ministered to these
> peoples.[1]

Adherents of the Black Legend argue that not only were the Spanish sadistic murderers, they also were notorious exploiters of human
labor under conditions that were so dangerous that they led to the
death of countless Amerindians. In the Greater Antilles, Indian men
were forced to travel vast distances to toil in the mines, while their
wives stayed at home and cultivated their cassava plots. When at last
able to reunite, at intervals of every eight to ten months or more,
"they were so exhausted and broken and ground down that they, [men]
and women, had little inclination for marital communication; in this
fashion they ceased procreation." The shock of conquest and the cruel
exploitation of the natives may have contributed to loss of the will to
survive. Not only did parents abstain from intercourse; they at times
resorted to infanticide to check the cycle of oppression. Las Casas
remembered, "The newborns died soon, because their mothers, because of the hardship and hunger, had no milk in their breasts. For
this reason, while I was in Cuba, 7,000 children died in three months.
Some mothers even drowned the infants from sheer desperation. Others, when they felt they were pregnant, took herbs to abort, so they
were expelled stillborn." The tragic end for the island Arawaks came

---

1 Bartolomé de Las Casas, *Historia de las Indias*, 3 vols. (México: Fondo de
  Cultura Económica, 1951), 2:206.

quickly, as Las Casas noted. He further mused, "And it is here that one has to contemplate what would have happened if this set of causes had coincided for the entire world, would not the entire human line have been wiped out in no time at all?"[2]

Were Las Casas the only observer to point out the ruthlessness of the invaders, then we might conclude that he was deluded or that he simply invented to promote his cause in defense of Indian rights. As a propagandist for the protection of the native American, he might have warped the truth when he thought it was necessary. The ultimate end, human justice, Las Casas and others of like mind might argue, justified the means. But other, contemporaneous observers also pointed out the malicious way the Europeans acted toward native peoples. Pedro de Alvarado, for example, left in charge of the Aztec capital, Tenochtitlán, in early May 1520 when Hernán Cortés marched to face his enemy Pánfilo de Narváez, ordered the slaughter of masses of unarmed religious celebrants in the temple. The carnage was terrible. Native informants who supplied oral testimony to Friar Bernardino de Sahagún report the havoc as Spaniards fell on the packed throng, cutting off arms and legs and disemboweling their victims in a slaughter that continued until virtually everyone was dead: "So great was the bloodshed that rivulets ran through the courtyard like water in a heavy rain."[3]

Farther south, Spanish slaving in Central America in the 1520s was especially costly in American lives. Licentiate Cristóbal de Pedraza, another Protector of the Indians and subsequently Bishop of Honduras, reported that Alonso de Solís had burned fourteen Indians in Canola, "which seemed to this witness the greatest cruelty in the world."[4] If Indians tried to escape during forced marches, they were hunted down and run through with lances; war dogs too were used here with evil effect. Rodrigo de Castillo, a royal treasury official, reported to the Crown in 1531 that Spaniards on the march from Honduras to Nicaragua torched several neighboring villages and ripped recently delivered babies from their mothers' breasts and tossed them to the ground. Furthermore, captured Indians were enchained and forced to march long distances; if they fell during the transport, their heads were cut

2 Ibid., 2:250–51.
3 Bernardino de Sahagún, *Conquest of New Spain* (Salt Lake City: University of Utah Press, 1989), pp. 76–77.
4 William L. Sherman, *Forced Native Labor in Sixteenth-Century Central America* (Lincoln: University of Nebraska Press, 1979), p. 45.

off to avoid wasting the time it would take to stop and unlock the shackles. "In Aguatega 200 Indians were punished: one-third of them were put in a large hut and burned to death; another one-third were torn to pieces by dogs; eyes were plucked out, arms were cut off, and other cruelties were practiced on the remaining one-third of the Indians."[5] Rodrigo de Castillo pointed out that the best dogs receiving special training to hunt and kill native Americans became especially valuable, and they were sought out by those undertaking new expeditions.

Brutality seemed especially excessive during some of the lesser campaigns. Pedro Mártir reported that during Vasco Núñez de Balboa's conquest of Panama "the Spaniards cut off the arm of one, the leg or hip of another, and from some their heads with one stroke, like butchers cutting up beef and mutton for market. Six hundred, including the cacique, were thus slain like brute beasts. . . . Vasco ordered forty of them to be torn to pieces by dogs."[6] Similar accounts abound for the subjugation of the land of the Incas. In November 1536, during the rising of Manco Capac, a Spanish force under Alonso de Alvarado left Lima to engage rebels in the Jauja district. One soldier, Juan de Turuegano, later wrote to an associate in Seville that "the Christians captured a hundred alive and killed more than thirty. They cut off the arms of some they captured, and the noses of others, and the breasts of the women. And they then sent them back to the enemy, so that they could see that any who wanted to continue rebelling could see that they also would have to submit to the knife."[7] Again, what caused such atrocities? Was it the heat of battle that led some to become almost inhuman, or was it fear that such a small number of outsiders would have to destroy the will of the enemy masses brutally in order to survive? But would the exigencies of warfare justify the atrocities committed?

Evidence presented by the Spaniards, especially by Bartolomé de las Casas in his polemical writings, and the reports of many others, either eyewitnesses or contemporary gatherers of hearsay, have provided more than adequate proof for generations to lay the blame for the catastrophic demise of Amerindians on the European conscience. The Spaniards were blamed for the quick disappearance of the peace-

5 Ibid., p. 46.
6 David E. Stannard, *American Holocaust. Columbus and the Conquest of the New World* (New York: Oxford University Press, 1992), p. 83.
7 Raúl Porras Barrenechea, ed., *Cartas del Perú (1524–1543)* (Lima: Sociedad de Bibliófilos Peruanos, 1959), p. 272.

ful island Taino, encountered by the Columbus expeditionaries in 1492. Within fifty years the original islanders were virtually extinct. Central Mexico's population fell from nearly 15 million in 1519 to 1.5 million a century later, and there was a similar demographic collapse of Andean America.[8] A century after first contact the regions least affected by the disaster lost at least 80 percent of their people, 90 percent or more was more typical, and some regions became destitute of people. Las Casas wrote that 20 million Indians died in the encounter; the actual number may be close to Las Casas's estimate.

But the cause of the disaster was more than Spanish cruelty. Amerindians died wherever Europeans trod. They succumbed following contact with the Portuguese, then the English, the French, and the Dutch. Substantial numbers of deaths continued, no matter which European territory was involved, regardless of the location of the region. It seemed to make no difference what type of colonial regime was created; those who lived in the mission territories under the supposedly benign and caring administration of friars seemed to die as rapidly as those subjected to forced labor in dangerous silver and gold production.

Stories of Spanish cruelty in the New World fit perfectly with the evolution of early modern-European nationalism. The *Apologetic History* of Las Casas was translated and reissued many times during the sixteenth century. The inclusion of the descriptions of Las Casas in the illustrated editions of Theodore de Bry gave reality to what one might characterize as Spanish sadism in the popular mind of the century. The translations of the important texts of exploration and discovery by the English, especially Richard Hakluyt, opened the eyes of others to the wealth and opportunities for profit, and at the same time proved that because the Iberians were so reprehensible, their own actions could be justified easily. In a similar vein the translated narratives of de Bry provided the French with insight into the Spanish successes, as well as their weaknesses, in the Americas.

An equally vivid European depiction of the tragedy of conquest is

8 William M. Denevan, ed., *The Native Population of the Americas in 1492*, 2d ed. (Madison: University of Wisconsin Press, 1992), provides an excellent survey, with bibliography, of the estimates of the size of the native population at contact. See also a special issue of the *Annals of the Association of American Geographers* 82 (1992), on the question of "The Americas before and after 1492: Current Geographical Research"; and Nicolás Sánchez-Albornoz, *La población de América Latina desde los tiempos precolombinos al año 2025* (Madrid: Alianza Editorial, 1994).

Girolamo Benzoni's account of the disappearance of the Indians of Hispaniola. His text, alongside the plates of Theodore de Bry, provides a compelling picture of events in the Indies. Both Benzoni and de Bry conveniently ignored disease; both were filled with anti-Spanish hatred and became part of the group that disseminated the propaganda that formed the basis of the Black Legend. Benzoni was born in Milan in 1519. In 1541, driven by the same forces that compelled some of his young contemporaries to search out the New World, he traveled to Medina del Campo, then Seville, and finally set sail from Sanlúcar de Barrameda for the Indies. He was in the Americas until 1556, traveling from the Caribbean into Mesoamerica, Peru, then back to Nicaragua. The first edition of Benzoni's book *La historia del Mondo Nuovo* was published in Venice in 1565; a second edition appeared there in 1572. Theodore de Bry, who became a staunch Protestant, was born in Liège in 1528; he fled in 1570 and settled in Frankfurt am Main. De Bry is better known as a publisher and engraver than as the bookdealer he became. The first volume of his *Great Voyages* was printed in 1590. By the time he died in 1598 six volumes had been published. His heirs continued to publish travel literature, enlarging the series to thirteen volumes in 1634. Almost all were filled with anti-Spanish propaganda. The illustrations provided to even the most casual reader a visual image of Spanish depravity and greed.

Benzoni wrote vividly of the terrible exploitation of native peoples and their loss of will. The inhabitants of Hispaniola came to "feel oppressed by intolerable and insufferable miseries that were brought against them, and they believed there would be no way to recuperate their liberty. Giving way to sighs and lamentations, they longed for death." The chronicle of the despair of the Amerindians that Benzoni provided has been used over and over by the detractors of Spanish hegemony.

> From here, many, giving up all hope, went into the woods and hanged themselves from the trees, having first killed their children. . . . The women, with the juices of some plants, interrupted their pregnancies, so as not to give birth, and then followed in the footsteps of their men, hanging themselves. Some threw themselves from a hilltop over a precipice; others jumped into the sea, or threw themselves into rivers, or starved themselves to death. . . . And in the end, concluding it, of the two million Indians that there were on this island, between those

who commited suicide and those who died victims of Spanish cruelty, there do not remain today even one hundred fifty thousand.[9]

Yet cruelty explains only part of the reason for the conquest and disappearance of the Amerindian. Even in the late seventeenth century the Guatemalan chronicler Francisco Antonio de Fuentes y Guzmán, in the *Recordación Florida,* so angered by the insistent claims of Bartolomé de las Casas that the Indians had died largely at the hands of the conquerors, pointed out to readers that the Dominican friar had failed to mention Old World disease. Born around 1643, Fuentes y Guzmán held secular positions in Guatemala and died in Sonsonate in early 1700.[10] Referring in his history to the probable measles epidemic of 1533 that swept Guatemala, he noted that by not properly taking into account the impact of disease for the demise of Amerindians, the close link Las Casas made between European cruelty and the disappearance of Indians is not entirely accurate.[11]

Careful review of the extensive work of Bartolomé de las Casas indicates that he too knew of the impact European disease was having on Indian peoples. The most widely read text by the friar, and the only book-length work of his published during his lifetime, the *Brevísima relación* was written by a man trained as a solicitor, and in it he presented his case in defense of the Indians whom he saw as being at the mercy of the Europeans. That book and the multitude of translations and foreign editions became the cornerstone of the Black Legend. His writings were used time after time by Spain's enemies to justify their own encroachments on Iberian territory. As he pressed the Crown and Council of the Indies for decrees to protect the Indians, he could not give, as a trained lawyer, a truly balanced account of all the reasons for their demise. Elsewhere in his voluminous writings, particularly his multivolume history of the Indies, he did acknowledge disease. For example, the 1518 smallpox epidemic that swept Hispaniola, the Caribbean, and beyond was brought on "by

9 Girolamo Benzoni, *Historia del nuevo mundo* (Madrid: Alianza Editorial, 1989), pp. 144–45.
10 Francisco Esteve Barba, *Historiografía indiana* (Madrid: Editorial Gredos, 1964), p. 281.
11 W. George Lovell, "Disease in Early Colonial Guatemala," in *Secret Judgments of God: Old World Disease in Colonial Spanish America,* ed. Noble David Cook and W. George Lovell (Norman: University of Oklahoma Press, 1992), p. 69.

the will or permission of God, in order to free the few Indians who remained from so much torment and the anguished life that they suffered from, in all types of labor, especially in the mines." Las Casas argued as well that the epidemic was God's way of punishing the Europeans who oppressed the native Americans. God had permitted disease and death to liberate the Amerindians from their sufferings.[12] Las Casas contemplated the multiple reasons for the disappearance of Amerindians, and although he attributed major losses to the excessive demands and greed of the conquerors, he also recognized that disease contributed to the rapid decimation of the native populations.

The guilt that Las Casas placed on the Spaniards incensed many of the friar's compatriots, even at the time. In 1555, Friar Toribio de Benavente, known as Motolinia, wrote a missive to his monarch Charles V to refute the arguments of the Dominican Protector of the Indians. Motolinia admitted vast population losses, two-thirds, or even seven-eighths in some districts of New Spain, but he offered as the principal cause the successive epidemics that swept the land, especially smallpox and typhus. Why did the Amerindians die so easily? He speculated that their earlier sins of drunkenness and idolatry might have led to retribution but admitted that it was impossible for anyone to fully fathom divine will. Nevertheless, the demise of Indian America should not be blamed on the settlers, as Las Casas had argued so vehemently.[13]

By the late sixteenth century, the Black Legend was the stuff of common belief of non-Iberian Europeans. The role of the Spanish Hapsburgs as the defenders of the True Faith against religious reformers to the north, and their frequent and willing use of the instruments of the Inquisition to search out heterodox beliefs, reinforced in the minds of many the idea that they were ruthless and bigoted. Philip II's attempt to invade England in 1588, and the subsequent efforts of the Iberian Hapsburg monarchy against Protestant nationalists in the Low Countries and Central Europe, compounded anti-Spanish feelings. If the Spanish were truly as barbarous and cruel as depicted in the popular literature, then any action taken against them in Europe or within their overseas territories could be justified. Reports of direct Spanish attacks against the newcomers, such as the massacres of the

12 Las Casas, *Historia de Indias*, 3:270–71.
13 David A. Brading, *The First America. The Spanish Monarchy, Creole Patriots, and the Liberal State 1492–1867* (Cambridge: Cambridge University Press, 1991), p. 189.

men of the fleet of John Hawkins at San Juan de Ulloa in 1563 and of the French Huguenots at Matanzas inlet on the Florida coast in 1565, reinforced ideas of Spanish brutality. The Black Legend was firmly rooted at the core of European nationalism by the late sixteenth century. It was commonly believed that the evils perpetrated on inno-cent and ill-armed natives by the Spaniards led to the natives' precipi-tous disappearance. There was no reason to invoke other causes, for there were available many "true" histories of destruction that had been written by the conquerors themselves.

The rhetoric changed little in subsequent centuries. The Black Legend was an accepted paradigm in non-Hispanic European commu-nities. There were peaks of Hispanophobia during periods of height-ened nationalistic fervor, and the main features of the Black Legend lingered well into the twentieth century. Anglo-Americans in the United States adopted the anti-Spanish biases of their motherland and carried them to a peak of jingoistic frenzy in the Spanish-American War of 1898. At critical junctures the dusty bottle of the Black Legend has been uncorked and its thick venom released with predictable regularity at each commemoration of a major anniversary of the histor-ical confrontation. In the twentieth century we have initiated a re-evaluation of the creation of the Black Legend and have searched for other causal forces to explain the conquest and collapse of Indian America. This reexamination has led to a realization that the caus-ative elements of the Black Legend cannot fully explain the demo-graphic collapse of Indo-America.[14]

There were too few Spaniards to have killed the millions who were reported to have died in the first century after Old and New World contact.[15] If more native Americans died as a consequence of disease than as a result of warfare, then we need to identify the sicknesses, date their first and subsequent appearances, and ascertain the rates of morbidity and mortality. It is impossible to factor out and weigh precisely each of the causes that led to the collapse of Amerindian society. We might ask, Did the Spanish lance lead to the death of 2 percent of the Indians, the arquebus 5 percent, the dog 12? What percentage succumbed at the hands of their mothers who chose for their infants death rather than a life of pain and anguish later? And

14 Angel Rosenblat, "The Population of Hispaniola at the Time of Columbus," in Denevan, The Native Population of the Americas, p. 45.
15 T. S. Floyd, The Columbus Dynasty in the Caribbean, 1492 to 1526 (Albuquer-que: University of New Mexico Press, 1973), p. 153.

what percentage were never born, because males and females, suffering profound "cultural shock," had chosen not to procreate? Unfortunately, these questions are not amenable to historical research; we can only surmise on the basis of incomplete and flawed evidence.

The breakthrough in understanding the ecological disaster afflicting the Amerindian came with the revolution in modern medicine. Although natural causes of illness were suggested by sixteenth- and seventeenth-century physicians, a fuller and more complete understanding of human disease and the nature of its dissemination did not come until the twentieth century. One of the first to look in a systematic way at smallpox and its horrible impact on Amerindians was John Duffy in 1951.[16] In a trailblazing survey, Duffy documented that smallpox was one of the major killers and that its medical conquest was amazingly slow despite knowledge of the mode of control provided by Jenner in the late eighteenth century. In the late 1960s, in a succinct essay, Alfred W. Crosby took the next step, linking pestilence and conquest, cogently articulating the disease factor in New World conquest. His subsequent work expanded the theme to include other illnesses as well as plants and animals, and it spatially extended the argument from the Americas to the entire globe. He argued that largely European peoples have profoundly modified the world's environment in a relatively brief temporal span coinciding with the age of exploration, conquest, and colonization, running from the sixteenth century to the present.[17]

Recent scholarship by Alfred Crosby and others such as Sherburne F. Cook and Woodrow Borah, Francisco Guerra, Enrique Florescano and Elsa Malvido, Henry F. Dobyns, Russell Thornton, W. George Lovell, and Thomas M. Whitmore documents the impact of Old World diseases on New World populations.[18] Indeed, after a compel-

16 John Duffy, "Smallpox and the Indians in the American Colonies," *Bulletin of the History of Medicine* 25(1951):324–41; idem, *Epidemics in Colonial America* (Baton Rouge: Louisiana State University Press, 1953).

17 Alfred Crosby, "Conquistador y Pestilencia: The First New World Pandemic and the Fall of the Great Indian Empires," *Hispanic American Historical Review* 47(1967):321–37; idem, *The Columbian Exchange: Biological and Cultural Consequences of 1492* (Westport, CT: Greenwood Press, 1972); idem, "Virgin Soil Epidemics as a Factor in the Aboriginal Depopulation in America," *William and Mary Quarterly* 33(1976):289–99; and idem, *Ecological Imperialism: The Biological Expansion of Europe, 900–1900* (Cambridge: Cambridge University Press, 1986).

18 For a succinct bibliography of new contributions to the field, see William M. Denevan, "Native American Populations in 1492: Recent Research and a

ling effort to simulate population loss caused by epidemic disease and taking into account many variables, Whitmore concluded, "Since epidemics can account for virtually all of the extra mortality in the sixteenth century, the principle of Occam's razor suggests that it is not necessary to assume that there were other important causes of death. Thus, no reliance on the 'Black Legend' of Spanish homicide and cruelty is necessary to explain the observed population collapse."[19] Despite the number of scholars who have combined in constructing a logical argument laying most of the blame for the demise of the Amerindian on microbes, the advocates of the theory that Spanish cruelty was the primary factor in the collapse of native empires have continued to press their arguments. From the 1960s into the late 1980s, Marxist or neo-Marxist students focused on the issue of exploitation as the key element of European control of native peoples and the deaths of those suffering under the yoke of colonialism. Indeed, T. S. Floyd at the time charged that "the issue of Spanish cruelty to the Indian seems to have acquired even more distortion in recent

Revised Hemispheric Estimate," in idem, Native Population of the Americas, pp. xvii–xxxviii; see also Francisco Guerra, "La epidemia americana de influenza en 1493," Revista de Indias 45(1985):325–47; idem, "El efecto demográfico de las epidemias tras el descubrimiento de América," Revista de Indias 46(1986):41–58; idem, "The Earliest American Epidemic: The Influenza of 1493," Social Science History 12(1988):305–25; Enrique Florescano and Elsa Malvido, eds., Ensayos sobre la historia de las epidemias en México, 2 vols. (México: Instituto Mexicano de Seguridad Social, 1982); Elsa Malvido, "Factores de despoblación y reposición de Cholula (1641–1810)," Historia Mexicana 89(1973): 52–110; Henry F. Dobyns, "An Outline of Andean Epidemic History to 1720," Bulletin of the History of Medicine 37(1963):493–515; idem, "Estimating Aboriginal American Populations: An Appraisal of Techniques with a New Hemispheric Estimate," Current Anthropology 7(1966):395–449; idem, Their Number Become Thinned: Native American Population Dynamics in Eastern North America (Knoxville: University of Tennessee Press, 1983); Russell Thornton, American Indian Holocaust and Survival. A Population History since 1492 (Norman: University of Oklahoma Press, 1987); W. George Lovell, "Disease and Depopulation in Early Colonial Guatemala," in Secret Judgments of God: Old World Disease in Colonial Spanish America, ed. Noble David Cook and W. George Lovell (Norman: University of Oklahoma Press, 1992), pp. 49–83; idem, Conquest and Survival in Colonial Guatemala: A Historical Geography of the Cuchumatán Highlands, 1500–1821, rev. ed. (Montreal and Kingston: McGill-Queen's University Press, 1992); idem, " 'Heavy Shadows and Black Night': Disease and Depopulation in Colonial Spanish America," Annals of the Association of American Geographers 82(1992):426–43.

19 Thomas M. Whitmore, Disease and Death in Early Colonial Mexico: Simulating Amerindian Depopulation (Boulder, CO: Westview Press, 1992), p. 208.

years than it commonly carried, having become entangled with racism, modern ideas of liberty, and other notions inappropriate to the historical context."[20] Even as the disease factor was more thoroughly analyzed and expounded, the proponents of cruelty pushed forward with missionary-like zeal. Briefly in the early 1990s, with the quincentenary of the Columbus encounter, it seemed that the advocates of calculated cruelty on the part of the invaders had the upper hand.[21]

Heated arguments persist, and there has been substantial, though admittedly slow, research by a community of scholars who have been quietly accumulating piece by piece data on early epidemics in the Americas and their relation to subjugation of native peoples.[22] Many investigators have examined elements of the process: Crosby stressed the disease component as one of many in the process of ecological change; McNeill evaluated the experience of the Americas as part of the overall relation of disease to global historical change; C. W. Dixon with Donald R. Hopkins and H. Zinnser separately evaluated the particular impact of smallpox and typhus.[23] But until now no work has sythesized the findings. A study of disease in early colonial Brazil might be hidden in an obscure journal in France. The findings on sixteenth-century Quebec may not be known to someone working on the early contact in Tierra del Fuego. My purpose is to bring together in a succinct volume what is currently known of epidemic disease, especially as it relates to the conquest of native America.

A new paradigm points to the unleashing of a series of deadly epidemics as the principal consequence of European expansion. Contagion began at various places in America, then spread outward largely by migration. Some groups were devastated; others were spared. But those who had first escaped were hit by later waves of disease. It is difficult to extract unequivocal proof to support the paradigm, for the

20 Floyd, *Columbus Dynasty*, pp. 152–53.
21 In this group I include Stannard, *American Holocaust*, and Ronald Wright, *Stolen Continents: The Americas through Indian Eyes since 1492* (New York: Houghton Mifflin, 1992).
22 Linda Newson, Suzanne Alchon, Kristin Jones, Shepard Krech, Thomas Whitmore, and Robert Jackson are just a few specialists making recent important contributions to the study of Amerindian disease and depopulation.
23 Crosby, *Ecological Imperialism*; William H. McNeill, *Plagues and Peoples* (Garden City: Anchor Doubleday, 1976); C. W. Dixon, *Smallpox* (London: J. and A. Churchill, 1962); Donald R. Hopkins, *Princes and Peasants. Smallpox in History* (Chicago: University of Chicago Press, 1983); H. Zinnser, *Rats, Lice and History* (New York: Bantam Books, 1960).

evidence is imperfect. There are many reasons for the ambiguity; one of the most important is the virtual impossibility of accurately identifying sixteenth- and seventeenth-century illnesses. Other than cataloguing the symptoms, which is subject to a wide range of variations in both the infected person and in the abilities of the observer who chronicled the case, we have no clinical record of which diseases swept the two worlds united by the Columbus encounter. No viral disease can be conclusively identified without an electron microscope, a medical tool unavailable until the middle of the twentieth century. Hence there is bound to be controversy about the nature and course of colonial outbreaks of disease. Furthermore, not all the closest observers – the clerics who so assiduously recorded deaths in parish registers after the Trentine Reforms – bothered to describe the causes of the demise of their parishioners. Most clerics were more interested in the spiritual hereafter than in a medically sound examination and recording of the symptoms of illness. Death was, after all, something that occurred at the time and in the manner willed by an omnipotent deity; men and women had little power to modify Providence. Physicians might have attempted to intervene in the processes of disease and dying, but there were few trained practitioners, and their cures often were secured by chance rather than application of sure medical knowledge.[24]

Debate, uninformed debate, is a necessary consequence of incomplete information. The century and a half after 1492 witnessed, in terms of the number of people who died, the greatest human catastrophe in history, far exceeding even the disaster of the Black Death of medieval Europe. Although the written evidence is scattered and imperfect, the historian does have information from diverse sources, from the codices of stilled voices of Mesoamericans to the oral traditions of Andean peoples that were passed from one generation to another by the pens of colonial administrators. We also have letters from settlers – sometimes even the treatises and letters of those who understood best, the physicians. Almost all sources provide confirmation that sickness made conquest and foreign domination easier, not just for the Spanish but for all European states. The second great Columbus expedition, where we begin our examination, was the first to unleash the tragic round of alien infection. From that moment, and

24 Francisco Guerra, *Historia de la medicina*, 2 vols. (Madrid: Ediciones Norma, 1982).

continuing beyond the introduction of yellow fever in the middle of the seventeenth century, disaster followed upon disaster in an almost unbroken series of waves that led to a drastic reduction of the population.

The catastrophe seemed too profound to comprehend. No wonder some clerics referred to the "secret judgments of God" to explain the phenomenon. The death and debilitation of the survivors contributed to the European success in dominating New World peoples for more than three centuries. The present volume focuses on the nature and impact of the best-known episodes of disease that buffeted the Americas from Hudson's Bay to Tierra del Fuego from initial contact between the two hemispheres to the mid-seventeenth century. There was no escape for Amerindian peoples. Whether it was in the cold of the winter straits of the St. Lawrence or the hot and dry expanses of the Great Plains in midsummer, or in the insect-infested and rainy lowlands of Colombia's Atrato basin, or in the windswept stretches of Patagonia, the Europeans carried unwittingly in their breath the germs of destruction. No wonder, then, that so many lamented in their tragic plaint, "We were born to die!"

CHAPTER ONE

In the Path of the Hurricane

DISEASE AND THE DISAPPEARANCE OF THE PEOPLES OF THE CARIBBEAN, 1492–1518

In all the island you will not find a corner without such mounds, in clear evidence of its former tillage and of an innumerable population.

Bartolomé de las Casas on Hispaniola

They are not working people and they very much fear cold, nor have they long life.

Michele de Cuneo, 1495

Christopher Columbus first described the Lesser and Greater Antilles as an earthly garden of paradise. Consistently, he wrote of sizable populations and ample resources. What is more, the people were easily induced to share their food, possessions, even their women, with the outsiders. Where fresh water was abundant, the Spaniards discovered sedentary populations of agriculturalists whose productivity seemed to surpass that of the most advanced farmers of the Guadalquivir basin of Andalusia. Their diets were supplemented by hunting small land mammals, birds, manatees, and sea turtles, and fishing, as well as gathering shellfish. There seemed to be no want, compared to the periodic dearth facing the Europeans during years of crop failure and famine. Larger settlements of the island Taino consisted of several large houses concentrated around a central plaza in villages of up to 5,000 inhabitants. They were politically organized into a series of confederacies. Columbus may have exaggerated the beauty and wealth of the first inhabitants he encountered on his route to the Orient, but given the archaeological evidence, it is clear that most of the islands had substantial populations. It is also indisputable that the arrival of Old World peoples in the Americas was a watershed event that resulted in an unmitigated series of ecological disasters for native America.[1]

Although scattered low coral and sand islands were uninhabited, and others had only a scant human veneer – for example, the Bahamas and Lucayos as first seen by the Europeans under Columbus in October 1492 – others, especially the larger mountainous islands of Puerto Rico, Jamaica, Cuba, and Hispaniola, supported significant concentrations of people. Exact population numbers have eluded us, for it is unclear if the island residents ever formally counted themselves, and the first Europeans provided only quick and very impressionistic glimpses of the magnitude of the population. By the time the Spaniards set out to count the Taino on Hispaniola, they already were engaged in slave-raiding expeditions to nearby islands and were importing Africans to replenish their weakening and diminished local labor force. By 1542, a half century after Europeans reached the Caribbean, the once numerous Amerindian people were virtually extinct. They left behind place names, foods, and agricultural techniques, as well as some ceremonial sites. Any Amerindian vestiges among contemporary Caribbean peoples can most likely be traced to ancestors introduced from the mainland at a more recent time.

The disappearance of the aboriginal peoples of the Caribbean was quick and set a pattern that was repeated time and time again elsewhere in the hemisphere. There is no simple answer for the demographic collapse, because what happened after 1492 is a complex historical process and the factors are multifaceted. Outright military conquest was one factor, and here a superior level of Old World technology was important. Furthermore, ships permitted the movement of men, supplies, and reinforcements. The steel weapons, the sharp cutting edges of swords and lances, the gunpowder for the arquebuses and cannons, devastated those who defended their lands using Stone Age technology. The effective use of well-trained war horses provided Europeans with quick mobility and massive power. The horse was exceptionally effective in the conquest of regions without large mammals, such as the Caribbean islands and Mesoamerica. Savage attack dogs were employed as well, causing fear and bloody devastation. The Europeans' conduct of warfare was incomprehensible to the island Taino, for to compensate for almost incalculable numeri-

1 Irving Rouse, *The Tainos: Rise and Decline of the People Who Greeted Columbus* (New Haven: Yale University Press, 1992); David Watts, *The West Indies: Patterns of Development, Culture and Environmental Change since 1492* (Cambridge: Cambridge University Press, 1987).

cal inferiority, the Europeans sought to shock their enemy by massive killing, attempting to exterminate New World adversaries. If Europeans were captured in battle, they plotted escape, rather than accept their fate. European arts of diplomacy and warfare were alien to the Amerindians. By securing native allies, the foreigners helped compensate for their small numbers. Foreign rule through puppet leaders was effective in areas with developed states. Yet the critical factor in the European conquest and collapse of New World civilization was disease, deadly illnesses that devastated native Americans weeks and even years before the foreigners were faced directly for sickness spread from one native group to another.

Understanding the disease environment of the Caribbean in the years immediately before and during the first decades of contact sheds much light on the question of what occurred elsewhere in the New World. That the Caribbean was not a disease-free paradise must be a given. Illness existed in the New World before the arrival of the outsiders, and people died from infections. Recent research documents that histoplasmosis and tuberculosis were prevalent in America before Columbus. Certainly there were leishmaniasis and Chagas's disease in supportive ecological niches. Fairly widespread amoebic dysentery and intestinal worms weakened individuals and led to premature death, and various rickettsial fevers carried by arthropods were passed on to humans. There were salmonella and bacterial pathogens such as staphylococcus and streptococcus.[2] Furthermore, nonvenereal treponema – endemic syphilis – was found throughout the Americas. Influenza weakened and killed New World victims. Arguments continue among specialists on pre-Columbian prevalence of malaria and yellow fever. Potential mosquito carriers may have been in America, but the deadly forms finally experienced after 1492 were the consequence of Old World introduction of new vectors.[3]

2 Thomas M. Whitmore, *Disease and Death in Early Colonial Mexico: Simulating Amerindian Depopulation* (Boulder, CO: Westview Press, 1992), p. 50.
3 William M. Denevan, "The Pristine Myth: The Landscape of the Americas in 1492," *Annals of the Association of American Geographers* 82(1992):369–85, provides a succinct evaluation of recent research into the state of health in pre-Columbian America. Authors of most of the twenty-seven chapters in *Disease and Demography in the Americas*, ed. John W. Verano and Douglas H. Ubelaker (Washington, DC: Smithsonian Institution Press, 1992) examine the issue as well. Indeed, for a quick review of the subject, with full bibliography, this work is essential. Although the spatial focus is on mainland North America, other regions of the New World are surveyed. Whitmore's *Disease and Death in Mexico* (pp. 50–51) provides a quick summary. See also Ann L. W. Stodder and Debra

The killer diseases that were not native to the Americas included smallpox, measles, bubonic and pneumonic plague, typhus, and chol- era – the last not introduced until the early nineteenth century. All these, except cholera of South Asian origin, existed in various parts of Renaissance Europe, particularly in the larger cities such as Paris, Florence, Genoa, London, and Seville. In the fifteenth century several of these diseases survived in endemic form, persisting just below the surface and exploding into full-fledged epidemics in periods of crisis. Mortality levels were frightening even for the Europeans when malnu- trition and overcrowding made them more vulnerable to the disease. Conditions of warfare provided an ideal climate for the spread of such diseases as typhus. The long siege of the Kingdom of Granada bred outbreaks of typhus in Spain in the late 1480s and early 1490s, and the exposure of Iberian soldiers in the Italian peninsula in 1493 and 1494 led to continued mortality. Even the more common communica- ble crowd diseases of measles and smallpox claimed substantial numbers of victims, especially children. The more infrequent the epidemic, the more damage it did when it swept through countryside and city.[4]

The island of Hispaniola provides an excellent example of the toll that epidemic disease could extract from Amerindian populations that had never experienced European infections. The island played a piv- otal role in the European discovery and colonization of the Americas; it was the site of the first Spanish settlement in the New World, La Navidad. That north-coastal town was settled by a mere handful of men whom Christopher Columbus left behind when he returned to Iberia in early 1493 to report his supposed discovery of a new route to the Indies. Within months, Columbus was to return to the Caribbean with a fleet of seventeen ships transporting a contingent of 1,500 men to embark on a major effort to colonize. The island saw the first Spanish mining efforts in the Americas and the introduction of Old

L. Martin, "Health and Disease in the Southwest before and after Spanish Contact," in *Disease and Demography*, ed. Verano and Ubelaker, pp. 55–73; and John W. Verano, "Prehistoric Disease and Demography in the Andes," in *Disease and Demography*, ed. Verano and Ubelaker, pp. 15–24.

4 For an excellent synthesis of the history and diagnosis of epidemic disease, with chapters prepared by subject specialists, consult Kenneth F. Kiple, ed., *The Cambridge World History of Human Disease* (Cambridge: Cambridge Uni- versity Press, 1993). See also Ramón Sánchez González, "Hambres, pestes y guerras. Elementos de desequilibrio demográfico en la comarca de La Sagra durante la época moderna," *Hispania: Revista Española de Historia* 51 (1991): 517–58.

World cane sugar plantations. During the next quarter century the island acted as the outfitting station for subsequent exploration and discovery in the Caribbean basin and nearby mainland coasts. Virtually every ship that entered the Caribbean anchored, if only briefly, at the port city of Santo Domingo, founded on the south coast of the island in 1496. Santo Domingo became the main point of New World entry for the Europeans, their plants and animals, their pests and pathogens. The historical demography of the island is a microcosm of the tragedy that was repeated relentlessly throughout the Americas.

ELUSIVE NUMBERS

Almost all the first Europeans to disembark on Hispaniola's shores were impressed by the beauty of its peaceable Taino people and the land's bountiful resources. Sailing eastward from Cuba, Christopher Columbus sighted the island on Thursday, 6 December 1492, and enthusiastically recorded in his log that "there must be many people in this region, since I have seen so many canoes."[5] Five days later he wrote, "I thought that there must be a large population. . . . [A]ll the land is cultivated."[6] He soon described the land as "the most beautiful thing I have ever seen."[7] Two days later he sent a small force into the interior that reached a village he reported to have more than 1,000 houses containing over 3,000 persons. His joy was unrestrained: "As to the country, the best in Castile in beauty and fertility cannot compare with this."[8] On 24 December he claimed that the island "is larger than Portugal with twice the population."[9] Such hyperbole is not surprising, for Columbus was the greatest real estate agent of all time and was doing his utmost to collect enough "evidence" to convince others of the profits to be made in future investments in voyages of trade and settlement.[10]

5 Christopher Columbus, The Log of Christopher Columbus, trans. Robert H. Fuson (Camden, ME: International Marine Publishing, 1987), p. 129.
6 Ibid., pp. 130–31.   7 Ibid., p. 132.   8 Ibid., p. 134.   9 Ibid., p. 155.
10 The mental state of Columbus has received attention from many scholars. See Felipe Fernández-Armesto, Columbus (New York: Oxford University Press, 1991), pp. 84–93; and A. Milhou, Colón y su mentalidad mesiánica en el ambiente franciscanista español (Valladolid: Casa-Museo de Colón, 1983). S. B. Schwartz, The Iberian Mediterranean and Atlantic Traditions in the Formation of Columbus as a Colonizer (Minneapolis: University of Minnesota, 1986), places Columbus's activities in a realistic mode. For a straightforward account of the Admiral's sailing ventures, any of several works by Samuel E. Morison remain valuable.

Although Columbus exaggerated the number of people living on the island, its population must have been dense enough for the first visitors to concur with his overall impression of the potential profits to be made in subsequent ventures. The account of Michele de Cuneo, a participant in Columbus's second expedition, and whose distin-guished family seat was Savona, west of Genoa, elicits a greater level of confidence than most reports. A well-educated man and a keen observer of the voyage and the people he encountered, Cuneo wrote to a friend, Hieronymo Annari (15 October 1495). He had learned that at the time the Europeans arrived, two major cultural groups already shared the Caribbean. The docile Taino (Arawaks) were con-centrated in the Greater Antilles, and at the eastern extreme were the warlike and cannibalistic Caribs, who probably originated along South America's north coast and were occupying the Lesser Antilles, gradu-ally increasing pressure on their more peaceful neighbors. Cuneo was impressed by the number of islanders, saying "they are innumerable and inhabit an extensive territory," and suggesting that the islands verged on overpopulation. As were other early European observers, Cuneo was shocked by the island Caribs' apparent enjoyment of human flesh. But his gruesome descriptions are tempered by his Re-naissance interest in explication, in providing a rational explanation for unthinkable repasts. Michele de Cuneo's analysis is reminiscent of Thomas Malthus a full three centuries later. The Italian saw war as an effective check on Carib population growth, reporting that they often went out on raiding parties lasting from six to ten years. "They stay so long, whenever they go, that they depopulate the islands. And should they not do that, those Indians would multiply in such a way that they would cover the earth."[11]

How could the numbers of Taino have been so large as to threaten overpopulation? Bartolomé de las Casas, who arrived at Hispaniola about a decade after Cuneo and toiled many years on the island, was impressed with the fertility of its soils and the diligent labor of its inhabitants. He wrote, "The fields they had were in mounds of earth [conucos] which are not readily removed by water or wind; in all the island you will not find a corner without such mounds, in clear evidence of its former tillage and of an innumerable population."[12] The

11 Samuel Eliot Morison, Journals and Other Documents on the Life and Voyages of Christopher Columbus (New York: Heritage Press, 1963), p. 219.
12 Bartolomé de las Casas, Apologética historia de las Indias, in Obras escogidas de fray Bartolomé de las Casas, ed. Juan Pérez de Tudela, 5 vols. (Madrid: Biblio-teca de Autores Españoles, 1957–58), 5:chap. 20. My emphasis.

conucos were planted with yucca, corn, beans, squash, and a variety of other native crops. Hunting and fishing provided other necessary nutrients. Carl Ortwin Sauer, a historical geographer who examined the Hispaniola case, stresses the productive capacity of Taino subsistence activities and their ability to sustain large populations. He cites evidence from 1517–18, in which Jeronymite friars, entrusted with the spiritual conquest of the native people of the island, reported to the monarch that the crop yield of Taino agriculture was high.[13] Las Casas, in writings that extended over a career of more than a half century, more than once commented on the number of people the Europeans found in early postcontact Hispaniola. The friar, Defender of the Indians, at one point guessed a figure of a little over 1 million. In another treatise near the end of his long career, he reported 3 million. David Henige provides a strong cautionary note regarding the accuracy of figures given by Las Casas and other sixteenth-century observers.[14] Yet the early clerical witnesses may have been more accurate than modern scientists give them credit for.

The exact number of people living on Hispaniola in 1492 cannot be known. Nor can the exact number of residents of Aztec Tenochtitlán when first seen by Hernán Cortés in 1519 be established. Nor can the magnitude of the population under Inca ruler Atahualpa when captured by Francisco Pizarro's forces at Cajamarca in 1533 be ascertained. Although modern demographers can agree on the magnitude of New York City's population, they find it impossible to arrive at the exact number of people. Social statisticians actually estimate the approximate population of New York on the basis of flawed federal censuses and incomplete vital statistics. Contemporary demographers attempt to secure accurate data but tolerate a degree of error. Historians, in contrast to demographers, find it difficult to accept statistical manipulation of unknowns. Sixteenth-century evidence is weak; observers guessed population size on the basis of observation and analogy with known sizes, such as comparison with Venice, Seville, Portugal. Sometimes, as with the distributions of Indians in *encomienda* (a grant of Indians), people were actually counted, but not everyone at every place, at least during the first half century of European action in the

13 Carl Ortwin Sauer, *The Early Spanish Main* (Berkeley: University of California Press, 1966), p. 69; from *Colección de documentos inéditos relativos al descubrimiento, conquista y colonización de las posesiones españolas en América y Oceanía,* ed. L. Torres de Mendoza, 42 vols. (Madrid, 1864–1884), 1:247–411.
14 David Henige, "On the Contact Population of Hispaniola: History as Higher Mathematics," *Hispanic American Historical Review* 58(1978):217–37.

Caribbean. Modern historians have evaluated the evidence from the early observers, some have manipulated counts to determine depopulation ratios, and others have even attempted to establish carrying capacities for Taino agriculture. The results are all only educated guesses of one type or another.

The size of the island of Hispaniola, shared in modern times by the Dominican Republic and Haiti, is approximately that of Portugal. The range of modern estimates of the island's pre-Columbian population extends from a modest 60,000 (Verlinden 1968, 1973) to Borah and Cook's (1971) massive eight million (they actually projected 4 million to 14 million). Rosenblat (1967, 1976) and Amiama (1959) calculated 100,000; Lipschutz (1966) established a range of from 100,000 to 500,000; Córdova (1968) postulated 500,000; Moya Pons (1971, 1987) calculated from 377,000 to 600,000 for early contact; Cook (1993) provides a range of 500,000 to 750,000; and British statistician Zambardino (1978) projected 1 million, with a margin of error of about 30 percent (see Table 1.1).[15]

The debate among modern scholars is often heated, and given the wide diversity of opinion it is not surprising that it is at times acrimonious. But barring the chance discovery of a lost census of the island's people, it is unlikely that one can come much closer to a true understanding of the population dynamics of Hispaniola than did a German settler, Nikolaus Federmann, a resident of Santo Domingo for a time in 1529–30 and 1531–32. Federmann dryly observed:

It is hopeless to speak of the natives or inhabitants of this land, because forty years have already passed since the conquest of the island, and . . . almost all are gone. . . . of five hundred thousand Indians or inhabitants of various nations and languages that existed on the island forty years ago, there remain fewer than twenty thousand living. A large number died from an illness they call the *viroles* [Federmann includes this word, having heard the epidemic referred to as *viruelas*, smallpox, by the Spanish], others have perished in the wars, others in the gold mines where Christians forced them to work against their nature, because they are delicate people, and poor workers.[16]

15 For an evaluation of these estimates see Noble David Cook, "Disease and Depopulation of Hispaniola, 1492–1518," *Colonial Latin American Review* 2(1993):214–20.

16 Nikolaus Federmann, *Historia indiana*, trans. Juan Friede (Madrid: Artes Gráficas, 1958), p. 29; for the German, I use *N. Federmanns und H. Stadens*

Table 1.1. *Hispaniola's estimated native population*

Source	Year	Estimate
Verlinden (1973)	1492	60,000
Amiama (1959)	1492	100,000
Rosenblat (1959, 1976)	1492	100,000
Lipschutz (1966)	1492	100,000–500,000
Moya Pons (1987)	1494	377,559
Cordova (1968)	1492	500,000
N. D. Cook (1993)	1492	500,000–750,000
Moya Pons (1971)	1492	600,000
Zambardino (1978)	1492	1,000,000
Denevan (1992)	1492	1,000,000
Guerra (1988)	1492	1,100,000
Denevan (1976)	1492	1,950,000
Watts (1987)	1492	3,000,000–4,000,000
Borah & Cook (1971)	1492	7,975,000

Note: From Noble David Cook, "Disease and Depopulation of Hispaniola, 1492–1518," *Colonial Latin American Review* 2 (1993):215.

It would be difficult to find a more balanced and perceptive analysis of the demise of Hispaniola's native people. Federmann's direct experience on the island was brief, but he was a curious observer and certainly asked early settlers about the nature of the island at the time of the first expeditions of Columbus. Federmann is not melodramatic; he merely points out that a "great number" had died from smallpox, "others" by warfare, and "others" still, by labor in the mines. Might there have been half a million island residents in 1492, as Federmann wrote? Lacking exact data, twentieth-centry scholars have failed so far to arrive at an estimate that is significantly more convincing than Federmann's guess in the early 1530s.

Although modern estimates of the contact population of the island vary so markedly, there is general agreement on the figures of the early sixteenth century. The 1508 population, as Miguel de Pasamonte reported, stood at some 60,000. Within two years, in 1510, according to Diego Columbus, it was 33,523. By 1514, about 26,334 Indians

Reisen in Südamerica 1529 bis 1555, ed. Karl Klüpfel (Stuttgart: Literarischer Verein, 1859). This citation is from page 10 of the German text. Friede does not translate *viroles* as *viruelas*, but suggests, here erroneously, that it may be the generic word for "pestilence."

remained, according to a "census" report. The numbers fell to around 18,000 in 1518–19, and by 1542 the native American population of the island was less than 2,000. Very early, the European settlers initiated importation of slaves from Africa and Indians from other islands to provide a labor force for the island's economy. Regardless of our inability to know the exact size of the contact population, the consequence of the European arrival in the Caribbean is the same. A half-century later there were virtually no Amerindian survivors of the human disaster that changed forever the landscape first described by Columbus in 1493.[17]

We have seen that one fundamental cause of the cataclysmic disappearance of the Arawaks, argued so strongly by the "Defender of the Indians" Bartolomé de las Casas, was cruelty. The Dominican friar wrote the heated *A Very Brief Relation of the Destruction of the Indies* (*Brevísima relación de la destrucción de las Indias*) in 1542. His purpose was to advocate the cause of the Indians in the Council of the Indies in order to procure new legislation to check the exploitation inherent in the early Caribbean version of the *encomienda* system. His treatise was published first in 1552 in Seville, without royal authorization. In the years immediately following 1578, the polemical work was translated into six other European languages. Most of these translations were supported by Spain's enemies. More than fifty editions of the treatise had been printed by the second half of the seventeenth century. With sensationalist illustrations, the international best-seller was used by Spain's detractors to justify their own encroachments on lands that Las Casas described as having been taken illegally and exploited inhumanely. Cruel exploitation in the mines and plantations, rape and pillage, and outright barbarity led, in the popular non-Hispanic mind of the sixteenth century, to the demise of "peaceable savages." It came to be commonly believed that young native men cut off their limbs rather than serve in the gold and silver mines or to labor in the fetid fields of cane. Desperate mothers aborted by using native medications, or they hurled newly born infants over cliffs to save them from the ruthless Spaniards. Amerindian men and women gave up hope, they lost even the urge to reproduce, in a terrifying example of culture shock. Whether this account was true in fact was unimportant, for a vast number of people accepted the friar's passionate treatise as a true testament of the Spaniards' heartlessness and cruelty.

17 Cook, "Disease and Depopulation," p. 216.

Virtually all evolving nation-states touching the Atlantic or Hapsburg territories in the heart of the European continent joined in this
sixteenth-century attack on Spain's empire, accepting the tenets of
what came to be known as the Black Legend. Their own self-identity
came to be linked with blind opposition to the Catholic monarchs
and the Hapsburg dynasty. The Dutch, English, French, and even the
Portuguese, who lived under a Spanish king from 1580 to 1640,
became fervently anti-Spanish. The expanding European nation-states
quickly came into direct competition in overseas ventures in the
Americas, Africa, and later the Orient. It is little wonder that the
Black Legend took such deep and persistent root in European soil, for
it provided one of the foundations of modern nationalism. Because of
this persistent anti-Spanish propaganda, the disease factor was largely
overlooked as the fundamental cause of the demographic collapse of
the New World paradise.[18]

But the human agony of the first great smallpox epidemic to hit the
New World was impossible to ignore, and even Bartolomé de las
Casas, in his less popular historical writings, noted it. Even while it
was happening, observers reported on the destructive reaping of the
aboriginal population. Disease is the concurrent explanation for the
demise of the island Arawaks. Historian Alfred Crosby characterized
the initial New World smallpox epidemic as "an epidemic whose
influence on the history of America is as unquestionable and as spectacular as that of the Black Death on the history of the Old World."[19]
Smallpox stripped away about two-thirds of the remaining native
residents of the island in just a few agonizing months.

The 1518 smallpox epidemic does not explain what happened to
the island's population or to the rest of the Caribbean basin in the
quarter century preceding that terrible event. A handful of experts
have argued for an earlier smallpox bout that took place around 1507.
David Henige could find no evidence of epidemics prior to 1518,

18 The literature on the relationship between Las Casas and the Black Legend is
   massive. For an introduction to the complex subject, see Charles Gibson, ed.,
   The Black Legend: Anti-Spanish Attitudes in the Old World and the New (New
   York: Knopf, 1971); Lewis Hanke, *The Spanish Struggle for Justice in the Conquest of America* (Boston: Little, Brown, 1965); David M. Traboulay, *Columbus
   and Las Casas: The Conquest and Christianization of America, 1492–1566* (New
   York: University Press of America, 1995).
19 Alfred Crosby, *The Columbian Exchange: Biological and Cultural Consequences
   of 1492* (Westport, CT: Greenwood Press, 1972), p. 42.

concluding that "the early arrival of epidemics needs to be argued on the basis of some sort of evidence. To produce the specter of epidemiological disaster merely as a *deus ex machina* to explain the otherwise unaccountable results of a chosen statistical procedure [Borah and Cook] simply fails to persuade."[20] In a careful exercise in historical sleuthing, Henige traced the origin of a totally falsified 1507 smallpox outbreak recently accepted by some scholars, but according to Henige, only the consequence of "an illusion created by accident and perpetuated by carelessness."[21] Henige searched in vain for other pre-1518 epidemics without success. But evidence exists, and it is truly convincing.

THE FIRST EXCHANGE

It was not the first small fleet of three ships under Christopher Columbus that transferred Old World diseases to the Americas. In fact, the accounts of the first Columbus expedition to the New World provide little information on sickness. In spite of the duration of the trip and the poor quality of the provisions, the men seem to have been remarkably free from illness, "no one had been sick or even had a headache on all three ships, except for one old man with a long-term problem with kidney stone."[22] Indeed, the first disease contact between the two worlds was far more deadly for the Europeans than for the Amerindians. Several of the people who returned on the *Pinta* and *Niña* to the Iberian peninsula in early 1493 likely were infected with endemic New World syphilis. Most paleopathologists now agree that the archaeological evidence for long-term and widespread syphilis infection in the Americas is persuasive. The causative agent, the bacterial spirochete *Treponema pallidum*, or variations, triggers venereal syphilis, endemic nonvenereal syphilis, pinta, or yaws. The type is seemingly dependent on the people, nature, and place of infection, and some form of treponematosis seems to be prevalent in all human populations.[23]

---

20 Henige, "On the Contact Population," p. 235.
21 David Henige, "When Did Smallpox Reach the New World (and Why Does It Matter?)," in *Africans in Bondage: Studies in Slavery and the Slave Trade*, ed. Paul E. Lovejoy (Madison: University of Wisconsin Press, 1986), p. 15.
22 William D. Phillips and Carla Rahn Phillips, *The Worlds of Christopher Columbus* (Cambridge: Cambridge University Press, 1992), p. 169.
23 Brenda J. Baker and George J. Armelagos, "The Origin and Antiquity of Syphilis: Paleopathological Diagnosis and Interpretation," *Current Anthropol-*

Spain's most illustrious sixteenth-century physician, Nicolás Monardes, suggested that the infection that swept Europe came with
captured Indians from Hispaniola who were displayed by Columbus to
the court, "of whom most came with the fruit of the land, that was the
bubas. The Spaniards began to converse carnally with the Indian
women, and the Indian men with Spanish women, and in such fashion
Indian men and women infected the Spanish, Italian, and German
armies," and because there was a truce with the French and communications at the time between the forces, the French camp came to be
infected too. According to Monardes, the Spanish at first thought they
had caught it from the French:

> So they called it the French sickness. The French thought that
> since it was in Naples and from those of that land they had
> caught it, they called it the Neapolitan illness. The Germans,
> seeing that they were infected through intercourse with the
> Spanish, called it the Spanish *sarna*, and others called it measles
> from the Indies, and with much truth, for the illness came from
> there.[24]

The unintended revenge of the Spanish was smallpox. In the first
third of the sixteenth century, the historian Francisco López de Gómara wrote in his famous description of the Cortés conquest of the
Aztec empire that the great Spanish pandemic was so damaging in
Mexico City that it was necessary to pull "the houses down to cover
the corpses." They called the malady *huitzahuatl*, or "great leprosy," he
continued, and subsequently used the date as a marker for the end of
an old era and the beginning of a new. "They counted the year from
it, as from some famous event." López de Gómara succinctly sums up
the attitude of many of his contemporary compatriots as follows: "It
seems to me that is how they were repaid for the *bubas* which they
gave our men."[25]

ogy 29 (1988):703–37; Mary Lucas Powell, "Health and Disease in the Late
Prehistoric Southeast," in *Disease and Demography*, ed. Verano and Ubelaker,
pp. 41–53.

24 Nicolás Monardes, *Historia medicinal de las cosas que se traen de nuestras Indias
occidentales que sirven en medicina* [1574, facs. ed.] (Seville: Padilla Libros,
1988), pp. 13r–v.

25 Francisco López de Gómara, *Cortés: The Life of the Conqueror by His Secretary*
(Berkeley: University of California Press, 1964), p. 205.

The Second Expedition

Medical historian Francisco Guerra was the first to focus attention on the possible introduction of Old World pathogens into the Caribbean by the massive second expedition of Columbus.[26] The fleet, with seventeen ships and 1,500 all-male colonists, departed Cádiz on 25 September 1493. The expedition reached the Gran Canaries on 2 October, and finally the island of Gomera around 5 October. On board were Old World plants and animals the colonists planned to nurture in the new environment. Perhaps most significant, according to Guerra, were eight sows, loaded on ship on the island of Gomera in the Canaries between 5 and 7 October. Michele de Cuneo reported, "We brought *pigs, chickens, dogs and cats*, they reproduce there in a superlative manner, especially the pigs. . . . Cattle, horses, sheep and goats do as with us."[27] Bartolomé de las Casas later argued that the eight sows were the progenitors of all those found in the Indies.[28]

Guerra notes that both men and animals on board quickly sickened. The voyage from the Canaries to the Caribbean was swift, and with favorable winds the ample fleet reached the Caribbean island of Dominica on 3 November, then sailed slowly toward their destination. They spent six days on Guadalupe and landed a contingent there. On 13 November a group disembarked on St. Croix in the modern Virgin Islands. On 18 November, the ships anchored on the coast of Puerto Rico to take on provisions, staying there until 21 November. They finally reached Hispaniola around 28 November, touching land near where the first expedition had departed a little less than a year earlier, at hastily constructed Navidad under the protection of chief Guacanagari, ruler of Marien.

Almost immediately the illness that had come with the fleet of the second expedition spread. The infection passed from sows to horses, and by the time the animals and passengers fled the ship as they

26 Francisco Guerra, "La epidemia americana de influenza en 1493," *Revista de Indias* 45(1985):325–47; idem, "El efecto demográfico de las epidemias tras el descubrimiento de América," *Revista de Indias* 46 (1986):41–58; idem, "The Earliest American Epidemic: The Influenza of 1493," *Social Science History* 12 (1988):305–25.

27 Morison, *Journals of Columbus*, p. 217. My emphasis.

28 Bartolomé de Las Casas, *Historia de las Indias*, 3 vols. (México: Fondo de Cultura Económica, 1951), 1:351. Las Casas says "ocho puercas"; one or more of the sows was obviously pregnant.

disembarked on Hispaniola that November day, virtually all were infected. Illness debilitated the Spaniards, and the highly contagious disease rapidly spread among native peoples as the foreigners fanned out across the island. Columbus himself became so weakened that he was unable to write for weeks. Hernando Colón wrote later describing his father's condition, "Not only was the Admiral too pressed for time to chronicle events in his usual way, but he also fell ill and therefore left a gap in his diary from 11 December 1493 to 12 March 1494."[29]

Navidad was quickly deemed to be inappropriate for a permanent settlement, and in spite of illness afflicting almost everyone, Columbus set out to begin construction of a new headquarters to the east, at a place named Isabela. The site seemed excellent at first, but the work was hard, and the laborers lacked their accustomed European food-stuffs. Las Casas described the tribulations vividly: "The men all of a sudden began to fall ill, and because of the little sustenance that was available for the sick, many of them began to die also, so that there did not remain a man among the hidalgos and plebeians no matter how robust he might have been, who did not fall ill from these terrible fevers."[30] Columbus and later Las Casas initially blamed the ill health of the settlers on the fact that the men were far from home and the food was alien. Furthermore, many of the colonists began to feel defrauded that they were not going to find the gold that was promised when they had set out from Spain. Although the Admiral did not escape falling ill, and took to his bed, he did write a report for the monarchs that was dispatched with a twelve-ship fleet under Antonio de Torres. In the report, dated 30 January 1494, Columbus apologized that more gold could not be remitted to his sovereigns; the amount was paltry because "the greater part of the people we employed fell suddenly ill."[31] Columbus did not identify the illness; there are mere hints of his diagnosis, and he implied that mortality might have been higher. "It would be also extremely inconvenient to leave the sick men here in the open air."[32] It seemed to make little difference where on the island one traveled, for "the greatest part of those who have gone out to make discoveries have fallen sick on their return."[33] At

29 J. M. Cohen, ed., *The Four Voyages of Christopher Columbus* (Baltimore: Penguin Books, 1969), p. 158.
30 Las Casas, *Historia de Indias*, 1:363.
31 R. H. Major, ed., *Christopher Columbus: Four Voyages to the New World, Letters
   and Selected Documents* (Gloucester, MA: Peter Smith, 1978), p. 72.
32 Ibid., p. 73.   33 Ibid., p. 74.

the same time, Columbus optimistically reported that the health of
the settlers could be restored. Indeed, "they speedily recover their
health."[34] He further pointed out that fresh meat would help. Columbus concluded, lacking a more accurate understanding of the sickness,
what many travelers to unknown lands long before and since have
believed: "The cause of the sickness so general among us, is the change
of air and water."[35] Columbus specified that Antonio de Torres was to
bring back with the next fleet raisins, almonds, sugar, and honey as
well as rice, foods long considered by Spanish physicians to have
therapeutic effects that could speed the cure of illnesses.[36]

The second expedition's principal physician Diego Alvarez Chanca
made valiant efforts to heal those who fell sick. In fact, Columbus
commended the doctor's efforts in the report directed to the monarchs:
"You will inform their Highnesses of the continual labour that Doctor
Chanca has undergone, from the prodigious number of sick and the
scarcity of provisions, and that in spite of all this, he exhibits the
greatest zeal and benevolence in everything that relates to his profes-
sion."[37]

Doctor Chanca sent a separate personal report to Spain by the
Torres fleet. The physician stressed the impact of the illness on the
first European settlers. So great was their fatigue, he noted, that "the
Admiral had at one time determined to leave the search for the mines
until he had first dispatched the ships which were to return to Spain
on account of the great sickness (mucha enfermedad) which had prevailed
among the men."[38] Disease reigned over the native population as well.
When the Antonio de Torres fleet departed from Hispaniola, "the
Admiral improved from his indisposition and illness" and decided to
conduct a brief survey of the island.[39] By the time he returned to
Isabela on 29 March 1494, conditions had markedly deteriorated: "He
found all the men very fatigued, because few escaped from illness and
death, and those that still remained healthy, as a result of the little
food, were flaccid." The food shortage became critical, and rations
were reduced time after time, with the result that more settlers fell ill
and died.[40] Unfortunately, when the second fleet reached the Indies,
they discovered that supplies loaded in Andalusia were damaged and
spoiled. Columbus blamed it largely on the negligence of the ships'

34 Ibid., p. 75.   35 Ibid., p. 76.
36 Phillips and Phillips, *Worlds of Columbus*, pp. 201–2.
37 Major, *Columbus: Four Voyages*, p. 90.   38 Ibid., p. 68. My emphasis.
39 Las Casas, *Historia de Indias*, 1:366.   40 Ibid., 1:376–7.

captains, but high humidity and heat on the island contributed to spoilage. Both food and medicines ran out. Conditions were so critical that they "would purge five with one hen egg and with a kettle of cooked chick-peas." Some brought their own medicines but not enough, "nor such that was necessary for so many, nor to suit all temperaments."[41] Furthermore, there was a lack of people to serve or care for the ill. Many died, "primarily of hunger, and without anyone to even give them a cup of water, and burdened with many painful aches."[42]

There is additional largely overlooked confirmation that not all was well as the seventeen ships of the second fleet sailed westward in the autumn of 1493. Detailed review of the logs, diaries, and correspondence of Columbus and other participants provides several notices of illness that afflicted both Europeans and native Americans. In early 1493, Columbus had carried back to Spain ten Indians he had captured during his initial voyage. They were *lucayos y haitianos* (Bahamians and Haitians) and were baptized in Barcelona; the Admiral's purpose was both to train them as translators and to demonstrate to the monarchs the nature of the people of the newly discovered lands. In spite of inadequate food and a difficult voyage to Spain in early 1493, all ten islanders survived. Seven of the ten reembarked with the Indies fleet as they left the Spanish coast on 25 September 1493. Unfortunately, only two of the seven Indians reached Caribbean shores.[43] Doctor Chanca, in a long letter to the municipal council of Seville that he transmitted through Antonio de Torres as Torres left Hispaniola in late January 1494, remarked on the plight of the Indian interpreters that of the seven who had embarked in Castile, five died en route, and the other two "escaped only by the skin of their teeth."[44] Surely the Spaniards made strenuous efforts to secure the well-being of the trained translators, for the Indians were critical to the success of the new venture.

Native American mortality is difficult to assess, because the Spanish took no accurate count and had no grasp of the true size of the island's population in 1494. Yet the rough ratio of deaths of the translators that returned to the island in late 1493 with the second Columbus

---

41 Ibid., 1:377.   42 Ibid., 1:378.
43 Salvador Brau, *La colonización del Puerto Rico* (San Juan: Instituto de Cultura Puertorriqueña, 1969), pp. 32–33.
44 Juan Gil and Consuelo Varela, eds., *Cartas de particulares a Colón y relaciones coetáneas* (Madrid: Alianza, 1984), p. 171.

fleet, five of seven, suggests the very high levels of mortality that illness could produce. There was a similar elevated mortality among the 550 Indian slaves Columbus shipped off to Europe in lieu of treasure with the twelve ships in the Antonio de Torres fleet in January of 1494, Michele de Cuneo wrote after he returned to Europe in 1495. He had participated with Columbus in the reconnaissance of Cuba and Jamaica (April–September 1494), and he lamented bitterly about how difficult the return passage to Spain had been. Starting out from Puerto Rico, everything seemed to go wrong. Then, nearing the Spanish coast, 200 of the Indians died. Cuneo, as did Columbus, blamed the change of climate: "I believe because of the unaccustomed air, colder than theirs." But when they arrived in Cádiz, "We disembarked all the slaves, half of whom were sick. For your information they are not working people and they very much fear cold, nor have they long life."[45] Malnutrition and dehydration may have been factors, because food and water ran low and provisions spoiled on the overlong voyage. Starvation weakened the intended slaves, and they fell quick victims to new sicknesses never experienced in the warm and relatively isolated Caribbean. We cannot tell what the exact diseases were, but as we shall see shortly, Spaniards too were dying in large numbers in the mid-1490s.

Sauer provides another diagnosis for the troubles faced by the European settlers of Hispaniola in 1494. Based on the evidence of Doctor Chanca's letter, Sauer noted: "Within four or five days a third of the people fell sick. The illness continued for several months and affected the greater part of the newcomers. Las Casas said that hardly a man escaped the terrible fevers, many died, and the mood was one of anxiety and sadness at being so far from home and in such circumstances. The long voyage in close quarters must have been favorable to the spread of *intestinal infection*, further aided by their close congregation in building the town."[46] Contemporary medical historian Francisco Guerra attributes the 1494 illness to influenza, or swine flu. We know the tragic consequences of the 1918–19 worldwide influenza pandemic, when the 20 million deaths from the malady exceeded combat casualties in World War I. Guerra notes the symptoms described for Hispaniola: "high fever, ague, prostration and great

45 Morison, *Journals of Columbus*, p. 227.
46 Sauer, *Early Spanish Main*, p. 76. My emphasis.

mortality, though those who recovered did not relapse." As the disease spread, natives "started to die in infinite numbers."[47]

The sickness or sicknesses that afflicted both Spaniard and native American in late 1493 broke forever the ecological isolation of the two continents. A focus of infection established on Hispaniola that year could easily have spread to the nearby islands, for Puerto Rico, Cuba, and even the Bahamas were easily within the sailing capabilities of native Americans. In fact, if influenza were active on board the fleet, it would have first been introduced into the Lesser Antilles, then Puerto Rico, for the ships stopped there long enough for initial transmission from European to Amerindian. Both the leaders and common Spaniards were ill during the first months of exploration and settlement. We noted that Columbus was too indisposed even to write for several weeks in early 1494. Nonetheless, he was well enough to set sail and attempt to map out the southern coast of Cuba, then part of Jamaica (April–September 1494), which he circled. The Admiral reported that Jamaica was "a happy land . . . all the coast and land filled with towns and excellent ports . . . infinite numbers of Indians followed them in their canoes . . . all the land is everywhere very populous."[48] Jamaica came under permanent settlement in 1509. Columbus continued and explored part of the Cuban coastline. His son Hernando later wrote that during the inspection of Cuba, the "Admiral was utterly exhausted both by poor food and because he had not taken off his clothes or slept in his bunk from the day he left Spain to 19 May, and at the time when he wrote this he had been sleepless for eight nights on account of *a severe illness*."[49] Columbus was particularly stricken as he toured the Jamaican coast, and he returned to the Spanish settlement via the south side of the island of Hispaniola. By the middle of September he reached eastern Hispaniola, then sailed northward. He continued to Puerto Rico but failed to record it in his log book, according to Hernando. "The reason for this was his exhaustion from the great hardships he had suffered and his weakness from lack of food. He was afflicted by a *serious illness*, something between an infectious fever and a lethargy, which suddenly blinded him, dulled his other senses and took away his memory."[50] Las Casas reports that

47 Guerra, "Earliest American Epidemic," p. 323.
48 Las Casas, *Historia de Indias*, 1:393–94.
49 Cohen, *Four Voyages*, p. 175. My emphasis.   50 Ibid., p. 185. My emphasis.

after Columbus returned to Isabela he "was five months very ill, at the end of which Our Lord returned his health, for there still remained much for him to do."[51] Historian Samuel E. Morison suggests that Columbus suffered a kind of nervous breakdown during these months, but the symptoms could reflect a variety of afflictions.

Rather than continuing exploration of the lesser islands, the group headed west to Isabela and reached it on 29 September 1494. "Here God was pleased to restore the Admiral's health, although the illness did not entirely abate for five months," or until January of the following year, 1495. Some scholars have attributed Columbus's illness to gout; more recently Gerald Weissmann (1986) suggests he may have been suffering from Reiter's syndrome. Phillips and Phillips agree that many settlers of the second expedition may have been stricken with this disease, which is "characterized initially by dysentery and later by arthritic conditions, especially of the lower joints; inflammation of the eyes, and even blindness; and a penile discharge. Its cause is a tropical bacillus named *Shigella flexneri*, and is spread by unsanitary food handling."[52] Attribution of Reiter's syndrome to Columbus is not impossible, given the long-term evidence on his state of health. Spanish medical writers of the sixteenth century referred to the original illness as the flux, and it was usually associated with poor sanitation in concentrations of people in military encampments. Many or even most of the members of the 1494 expedition, as well as the Taino population, could have suffered from one or another form of bacillary dysentery. *Shigella flexneri* is just one type of several. All have in common a widely distributed bacterial agent that attacks the mucosa of the large intestine, resulting in dysentery. Incubation is one to four days, and onset can be sudden. The course of the infection described in a modern text resembles testimony provided by Dr. Chanca and Cuneo: "fever, drowsiness or irritability, anorexia, nausea, abdominal pain, tenesmus, and diarrhea. Blood, pus, and mucus appear in the diarrheal stools within 3 days." Severe diarrhea can cause dehydration, and death may come within twelve days of onslaught. Recovery can take up to six weeks.[53]

51 Las Casas, *Historia de Indias*, 1:397.
52 Phillips and Phillips, *Worlds of Columbus*, p. 200; Gerald Weissmann, "They All Laughed at Christopher Columbus," *Hospital Practice* 21 (15 January 1986): 30–41.
53 K. David Patterson, "Bacillary Dysentery," in *Cambridge World History of Disease*, ed. Kiple, p. 605.

Sickness continued. Antonio de Torres was able to return to Hispaniola in October 1494; he carried new supplies and fresh venturers.
He remained in the Indies briefly and sailed back to Spain in February
1495. In March Christopher Columbus captained a military force and
set out from the town of Isabela in company with the Taino chief
Guacanagari. During Columbus's extended reconnaissance of Cuba
and Jamaica, Spaniards on Hispaniola had so alienated the Taino that
they reacted violently against the settlers. In one case, "the cacique of
Magdalena, whose name was Guatigana, killed ten Christians and
secretly ordered the firing of a house in which *forty men lay sick.*"[54]
Columbus planned to punish those Taino who opposed Spanish rule
with such severity that future rebellion would be futile. Columbus
reported that the Spanish were greatly outnumbered; they faced some
100,000 Indians with only 200 Christians, twenty horse and about
twenty ferocious attack dogs. The Europeans believed that Divine
Providence intervened to save them. Columbus boasted that "he
thought it impossible that 200 men, ill-armed and half of them sick,
would have been sufficient to conquer such a multitude."[55] Columbus
was thankful that the native defeat was followed by a period of peace,
so that the 630 mostly sick Spaniards on the island at the time, a
number that by 1495 included women and children, were able to
travel about freely without fear of reprisals. Yet the Christians had
also suffered. Columbus believed that during these months God "had
inflicted on the Christians shortage of food and severe illness, which
reduced them to a third of their former strength."[56]

As often happens, starvation coincided with disease, and it affected
both Europeans and native Americans. According to Pedro Mártir de
Anglería, Columbus was informed by the natives "that there was such
a famine among the islanders that more than fifty thousand men had
already died, and they fall sick each day, at each interval, as livestock
from an infected flock."[57] According to Mártir, the primary cause for
the famine was human; the natives had decided the best way to be
delivered from the outsiders was to destroy their food, so they dug up
crops already planted and fled to the hillsides. But it is also likely that
the natives suffered from epidemic disease to such an extent that they
were unable to tend their crops. Famine is a regular consequence of

54 Cohen, *Four Voyages*, p. 187. My emphasis.   55 Ibid., p. 191.   56 Ibid.
57 Pedro Mártir de Anglería, *Décadas del Nuevo Mundo* (Buenos Aires: Editorial
    Bajel, 1944), p. 45.

epidemic disaster, and epidemics often follow on the heels of a major crop failure.[58]

The Crown was fully aware of the chaotic state of the island's affairs and sent Juan de Aguado to conduct a review of the Columbus administration. Aguado left Spain in October 1495, with three ships and approximately thirty settlers and much-needed supplies. Other fleets came; in July 1496 three ships captained by Peralonso Niño reached Isabela with more materials. But in 1497, no ship arrived from Spain.[59] Columbus's return to Spain from the second expedition was a near disaster; on 10 March 1496 the group with Juan de Aguado embarked from Isabela, transporting 225 Christians and 30 Indians on board two modest caravels. They sailed eastward, passing out of sight of the island on 22 March, but they faced strong headwinds. Getting nowhere and running short of provisions, they returned to Guadalupe.[60] There they landed and managed in a skirmish to steal a twenty-day supply of cassava bread and water from the Indians, and captured as well a female cacique and her daughter. They renewed their homeward trek again on 20 April. Unfortunately, at this point Columbus the pilot miscalculated, heading in a predominantly east, northeasterly direction. Too far in the middle of the Atlantic, and approaching what is today named the Bermuda Triangle, it was impossible to take advantage of favorable winds and currents, and the ships were too frequently becalmed. By 8 June, when the crew first sighted land somewhere between Lisbon and Cape San Vicente, the voyagers were desperate for food. By that time some of the Spaniards were proposing either to eat the Indians or to throw them overboard to lighten the ships. When the emaciated travelers finally disembarked in Cádiz on 11 June 1496, many had "the faces the color of lemon or saffron." Various historians have attempted to diagnose the problem, with varying results. Jarcho suggests that quite probably the entire fleet suffered from severe jaundice by the time they reached port.[61] Phillips and Phillips suggest that the coloration and weakness came "perhaps from

---

58 John Walter and Roger Schofield, eds., *Famine, Disease and the Social Order in Early Modern Society* (Cambridge: Cambridge University Press, 1989).

59 T. S. Floyd, *The Columbus Dynasty in the Caribbean, 1492 to 1526* (Albuquerque: University of New Mexico Press, 1973), pp. 30–33.

60 Cohen, *Four Voyages*, p. 195.

61 Morison, *Journals of Columbus*, pp. 250–51; Saul Jarcho, "Jaundice During the Second Voyage of Columbus," *Revista de la Asociación de Salud Pública de Puerto Rico* 2(1956):24–27.

tainted seafood."[62] Morison provides another alternative diagnosis, suggesting that many of the men probably were suffering from hepatitis.[63] The true explanation may be simple. Sebastián de Covarrubias Orozco, the compiler of the first modern Spanish dictionary (1611), provides one definition of "yellow" (*amarillo*) as: "Among the colors it is taken for the most unfortunate, because it is [the color] of death, and of a long and dangerous illness."[64] The emaciated passengers leaving the ship were described as yellow, the color of death, for they neared its final grip, most likely from starvation.

Disease felled both Amerindian and foreigner in the critical 1494–96 period. The Dominican friar Bartolomé de las Casas lamented that along with the second expedition of Columbus, there "came among them such illness, death and misery, that of fathers, mothers and children, an infinite number sadly died. Such that with the massacres of the wars and by the starvation and sicknesses that come because of them, and of the fatigues and oppressions that afterward took place, and miseries, and above all the great intimate pain, anguish and sadness, there did not remain of the multitudes of peoples that were on this island from the year of 1494 until that of 1496, it is believed, the third part of all of them."[65]

Massive deaths winnowed aboriginal Hispaniola and pared its foreign settlers between 1493 and 1496. It is evident from the contemporary descriptions that sickness with resultant high mortality, extended convalescence, and common relapses characterized the initial years of Hispaniola's full integration into the Atlantic world. Sickness was made more acute by failure of foodstuffs and the resulting starvation, by contaminated food and water, and by primitive hygiene. Francisco Guerra's assertion that the Spaniards unwittingly carried and introduced swine influenza seems plausible, but it is also possible that other diseases contributed to elevated mortality. Typhus, often associated with troop movements and warfare, was prevalent in Andalusia these years. The fall of Granada was accompanied by deadly typhus, and it lingered in endemic form. A severe strain of bacillary dysentery might also have caused the substantial loss of life during this period.

62 Phillips and Phillips, *Worlds of Columbus*, p. 211.
63 Samuel Eliot Morison, *The European Discovery of America. The Southern Voyages, 1492–1616* (New York: Oxford University Press, 1974), p. 138.
64 Sebastián de Covarrubias Orozco, *Tesoro de la lengua castellana o española* (Madrid: Editorial Castalia, 1994).
65 Las Casas, *Historia de Indias*, 1:419–20.

Prodigious numbers of deaths coincided with the second Columbus expedition, the consequence of starvation and epidemic disease. On the side of the Europeans, more than half of the 1,500 first settlers perished before Columbus returned to Spain. Of the Taino natives, untold numbers perished. Isabela, founded in early 1494, was one of the first ghost towns in the American experience of Old World peoples. It was abandoned not long after the city of Santo Domingo was established. Isabela's demise was linked to the high number of young Spanish dead during its first months of settlement, and there evolved around the site a feeling of desolation and anguish. Bartolomé de las Casas visited its ruins a little over a decade after it had become overgrown with underbrush. Las Casas wrote that it was commonly believed "that one did not dare to venture through Isabela after it became uninhabited without fear and danger, for it was said that anyone who had to pass by, or do something there, as those who came to herd swine, as well as others who lived in the fields nearby, would daily and nightly see and hear many fearful and horribly frightening voices. Because of this no one would dare to go there." Already there had evolved a legend that frightened locals as well as outsiders who came to see the abandoned settlement. The Dominican Protector of the Indians remembered that "one time one or two men came during the day into the buildings of Isabela. In one street there appeared two rows of men, in the fashion of two choirs. All of them seemed to be noblemen and courtiers, well dressed, wearing their swords and covered up in traveling hoods, of the type then used in Spain." Indeed, most of the men of the second expedition expected to find riches, not hunger, starvation, disease, and a shallow grave. The men "had so recently arrived and were so finely decked out, yet no one on this island had known anything about them." Perhaps here is a recollection of the remnants of the Amerindians who still managed to survive. They saw the intruders as well dressed, and the intruders did represent the cream of the young hidalgos of Iberia. But the Taino did not know who the outsiders were. "They greeted them and asked them when and from where they had come, and they responded without saying a word. Only, taking their hand to their hats as if to return a salute, along with their hats they removed the heads from their bodies, remaining headless, and then they disappeared." The mytho-historic perception was that many prosperous-looking foreigners had come to the land but had quickly died, leaving no recollection of even their names. "Those who had seen them were almost frightened to death from the vision and perturbation, and were tormented and terrified many days afterwards."[66] (See Map. 1.1.)

THE THIRD EXPEDITION

When Christopher Columbus sailed back to Spain in 1496, he left his brother Bartolomé in charge of the administration of Hispaniola. When the Admiral returned with a third expedition, it is likely that another set of Old World pathogens was introduced into the Americas. The fleet of six ships left Sanlúcar de Barrameda on 30 May 1498 and landed at the town of Funchal on Madeira, staying there six days to take on water and provisions. On 16 June they left the Madeiras and continued to Gomera in the Canaries. From here Columbus sent three ships ahead to Hispaniola with supplies. Here too the crew took on water, wood, and especially cheese, which was abundant on the island and was known for its excellent quality. Columbus continued to the Cape Verde islands, stopping at the leper colony of Boavista on 27 June. The settlement included only six to seven stone houses, although there were numerous goats. Here the explorers loaded salt and meat. On June 30, they continued to Santiago, where, according to the abstract of the journal made by Las Casas, "he wanted to take on some cattle to transport to Hispaniola, as the monarchs had commanded him. Accordingly, he stayed there eight days. But the Admiral was unable to carry out his orders. He reported that the island was most unhealthy, and that his men suffered from the heat and *began to fall sick*, he therefore decided to depart."[67] Columbus does not describe their sickness. Was it heat prostration, exhaustion, contaminated water, or something else? Whatever the case, the Admiral continued the voyage on 4 July, reportedly suffering gout and insomnia while sailing westward.

On the last day of July the fleet sighted the island of Trinidad. The following day the ships anchored, and crews on all three vessels landed to take on fresh water. They reported that there were farms, "and many villages"; the "land was well populated and cultivated." On 8 July they sailed along the Venezuelan coast, finding, according to Columbus, "innumerable houses and people . . . countless canoes. . . .

66 Ibid., 1:378.   67 Morison, *Journals of Columbus*, p. 262. My emphasis.

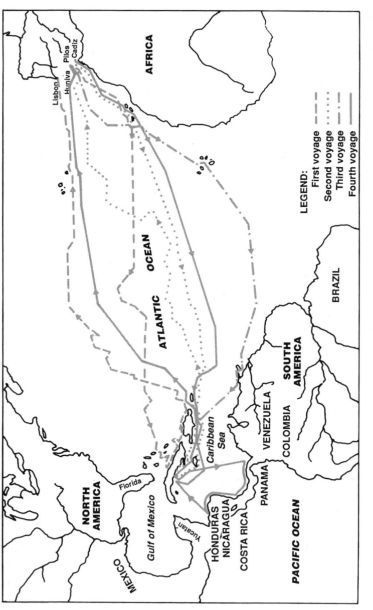

Map 1.1. The four voyages of Columbus. From William D. Phillips and Carla Rahn Phillips, *The Worlds of Christopher Columbus* (Cambridge: Cambridge University Press, 1992), p. 2.

[The people] are much more civilized than those of this Hispaniola
. . . the houses are attractive."[68] This region became in the early years
of the next century the source of Indian slaves taken to replace
Hispaniola natives. Licentiate Alonso Zuazo, who subsequently traveled to Hispaniola to conduct a *residencia*, or review of local administration, said that by 1518, some 15,000 Venezuelan Indians had been
taken as slaves to the island.[69] From the north coast of South America
the third fleet sailed northward and finally landed at Santo Domingo
on 31 August 1498. Columbus was in very poor health during the last
part of the voyage. His eyes were bloodshot, he could not sleep, or else
he would not, and he stopped writing, "on account of his *grave illness*
at this time."[70] Again the Admiral seemed to approach blindness.

The Europeans left on Hispaniola did not fare well during the
Admiral's absence. Around 1 July, the three caravels dispatched under
Peralonso Nīno arrived from Spain with needed provisions: wheat,
olive oil, wine, salt pork, and beef.[71] But the supplies, welcome as they
most certainly were, proved insufficient, and the settlers remained
discontented. The capital had been transferred from Isabela to Santo
Domingo, and there was growing exploitation of Indians that contributed to increasing rage against the Europeans. Health conditions were
poor; 300 Spaniards had already fallen victim to various unspecified
illnesses. They lacked medications and food, and they finally decided
it would be best to distribute settlers around the island in hastily
constructed forts.[72]

Inauspiciously, Christopher Columbus had left Francisco Roldán as
alcaide (chief warden, or governor of a fortress) and Justicia Mayor of
Isabela. Chafing against the rule of the Columbus family, Roldán
captained a group of disgruntled settlers and marched with supporters
from Isabela to take Fort Concepción in May 1497.[73] The revolt
sputtered on until the summer of 1499, when Roldán was finally
captured by Bartolomé Columbus. Yet the malcontents continued
their opposition to Columbus's rule, and from Santo Domingo Francisco Roldán wrote the Archbishop of Toledo on 10 October 1499 to
defend his actions, describing the terrible conditions that had faced
settlers the preceding year, 1498. He too mentioned illness: "At that
time the greatest part of the Christian people were sick of this general

68 Ibid., p. 271.   69 Floyd, *Columbus Dynasty*, p. 172.
70 Morison, *Journals of Columbus*, p. 279. My emphasis.
71 Mártir, *Décadas*, p. 52.   72 Ibid., pp. 54–55.
73 Floyd, *Columbus Dynasty*, p. 36.

illness that is going around." But there was not only sickness; due to insufficient rainfall the crops failed, and there was a great need for foodstuffs. Roldán complained that as he lay ill in Isabela the natives had taken advantage of Spanish weakness to rise and attack, killing "the Christians who were ill and scattered in many places, and without healthy men to stand guard."[74] Roldán learned that the garrison of Concepción was in jeopardy, for the Indians planned to rebel, and there were only eight men stationed at the post, "all sick (dolientes)." Roldán claimed to have prepared defense, concentrating there the sick people from all the neighboring estates. "They were dying of hunger, and there was nothing one could do about it." Several historians label this illness syphilis. Juan Gil and Consuelo Varela argue that "thirty percent of the inhabitants were stricken by syphilis."[75] It is likely that the attribution of syphilis by some scholars stems from Oviedo, who wrote about the loss of life at Isabela and the quickly abandoned garrison of Santo Tomás. He related that half of the Spaniards died of hunger and a disease that he described as a malady of pustules. Davies agrees that Santo Domingo was infected at the time: "More than 160 were sick with the French sickness [syphilis]." He suggests the most unlikely possibility that Spanish women sent from Castile actually carried the malady.[76]

It was during this period that members of a set of so-called Andalusian voyages reached the central Caribbean, bringing additional Old World pathogens. From about 1497 to 1501, several minor voyages from Southern Atlantic Spain led directly to a rapid expansion of the Europeans' geographic knowledge of the American land mass and contributed directly to the exchange of pathogens. In mid-1499 Alonso de Ojeda, with Amérigo Vespucci and Juan de la Cosa on board, touched the north coast of what became Brazil, perhaps discovering the mouth of the Amazon River. In September Ojeda and his men would land in the province of Xaragua in southern Hispaniola, and complicate the administration of Columbus. In November 1499 Vicente Yáñez Pinzón led a fleet of four ships out of southern Spain, and Diego de Lepe, commanding two ships, left just a few days later. The Yáñez Pinzón group probably briefly ascended the Amazon; Lepe and his men sailed farther west on the South American mainland

---

74 Gil and Varela, Cartas a Colón, p. 271.   75 Ibid., pp. 270–72.
76 Hunter Davies, In Search of Columbus (London: Sinclair-Stevenson, 1991), p. 218.

and discovered the Orinoco River. The Lepe fleet returned via the island of Puerto Rico, carrying a handful of slaves that his men had captured in the Orinoco basin. Yáñez Pinzón set foot on Hispaniola in June 1500. Both Yáñez Pinzón and Lepe lost men in combat with native Americans on the coast of South America. Some of the men in the combined fleets had been on the third Columbus expedition. The results of their discoveries would be shown on the famous 1500 world map prepared by cartographer Juan de la Cosa. All three preceded the "official" Portuguese "discovery" of Brazil by Cabral in 1500. Lepe secured authorization for a new voyage in 1501, but it is not clear if he was able to follow up. In a voyage of 1500–01, Alonso Vélez de Mendoza of the port of Moguer sailed southward along the Brazilian coast to encounter the Rio de la Plata estuary. The minor Andalusian discoveries concluded with the trip of Rodrigo de Bastidas to the Gulf of Urabá in 1500–1501.[77]

To argue that no disease transfer took place on these voyages is to assume the highly improbable. No efforts were made during the initial sailing ventures to block the flow of disease pathogens. Indeed, fifteenth-century Europeans lacked the medical knowledge to prevent the spread of potentially harmful organisms from one part of the globe to another. Medical practitioners in Seville realized that quarantine might, if they were fortunate and the block effective, prevent the arrival of the plague, which was about the only sickness that elicited such a forceful response. Thus, European diseases were loaded on board the ships tied up on the quays as surely as they were carried in the lungs, blood, and bile of the infected crew.

By the turn of the century, as a result of Columbus's chaotic administration of the island of Hispaniola, King Ferdinand and Queen Isabella named an agent to investigate and report on conditions in the Indies. Inspector Francisco de Bobadilla's modest fleet, including six Franciscans (Juan de Trasierra, Juan de Robles, Francisco Ruiz [a majordomo of Cardinal Cisneros], and Frenchmen Juan de Leudelle and Juan de Tisin, along with the chaplain, Benedictine Alonso del Viso) and a small number of settlers, left Spain in June 1500 and arrived in Santo Domingo in August 1500. Diego, Bartolomé, and

77 Juan Manzano Manzano, *Los Pinzones y el descubrimiento de América*, 3 vols. (Madrid: Instituto de Cooperación Iberoamericana, 1988), 1:291–311, 393–408, 429–33, 503; 3:52–55; Francisco Morales Padrón, *Andalucía y América* (Seville: Ediciones Guadalquivir, 1988), pp. 7–71; Fernández-Armesto, *Columbus*, pp. 145–6.

Christopher Columbus were arrested in October and placed on board a ship in the harbor. Columbus and Bartolomé suffered the indignity of being dispatched to Spain in chains, and a damaging report of Columbus's rule over the island was prepared.[78] The fleet set sail under captain Andrés Martín and reached Cádiz on 20 November 1500.[79] The Franciscans who had come to Hispaniola with Bobadilla soon posted letters to their superiors outlining conditions on the island. The set of complete papers concerning the Bobadilla *residencia* was lost or destroyed in a hurricane that sank most ships in a large fleet that set out on the return voyage to Spain two years later in July 1502, but we do have letters of three of the Franciscan friars who searched the island for converts. Friar Juan de Leudelle of Picardy wrote to Cardinal Cisneros in October 1500 that "we arrived at the island very well. Although to either a lesser or greater extent, we all tested the effects of fevers, in such fashion that when the caravels departed, we were already all well, except Friar Rodrigo and I, who are still not free of them."[80] He referred to the ill health of Friar Francisco Ruiz and others. In a letter dated 12 October 1500, Friar Juan de Robles reiterated much of what Leudelle had reported and argued that more missionaries were required, for already more than 3,000 Indians had been baptized. He noted that the land was extensive and the population large. Robles also related that the friars suffered ill health: "All of us became ill, some more, others less." He added, "Here one finds oneself always somewhat ill."[81]

From late 1493 to 1500 there are frequent references to sickness and food shortages on Hispaniola, initially extolled as an island paradise. The Europeans were obviously most interested in describing how illness afflicted their compatriots, not the native Americans. "Fevers" is most frequently listed as a symptom, with lethargy following. The most devastation may have taken place in early 1494, and the initial epidemic may well have been, as Guerra suggests, swine flu. But influenza accompanied malnutrition, especially among the Europeans, whose diet was inadequate in the first place and who found it extremely difficult to adjust to native American foodstuffs. Spanish mortality, caused by illnesses and outright starvation, may have approached two-thirds during the initial decade on Hispaniola. The native Taino mortality must have been even greater. For these conclu-

---

78 Floyd, *Columbus Dynasty*, p. 45.   79 Cohen, *Four Voyages*, p. 277.
80 Gil and Varela, *Cartas a Colón*, pp. 286–87.   81 Ibid., p. 288.

sions, we have only the impressionistic arguments of Pedro Mártir, who wrote that 50,000 men had already become ill at Hispaniola and that two-thirds had succumbed.

OVANDO AND THE 1502 SERIES

The massive fleet of newly appointed Governor Nicolás de Ovando transported many more settlers and potential illness to the central Caribbean. Ovando secured appointment for a two-year term; he would serve seven. He was charged to conduct the residencia of Francisco de Bobadilla and to prepare a thorough examination of the Roldán uprising. Composed of thirty ships, carrying 2,500 men and women, many of whom were Extremadurans from in or around Cáceres and Trujillo, the Ovando fleet sailed from Sanlúcar de Barrameda in February 1502. One ship was lost near the Canaries, and the fleet separated during the Atlantic crossing; they reached Santo Domingo in April 1502. They had departed from southern Spain during months that witnessed much hunger and sickness there.

Las Casas was one of the members of the group, and his firsthand testimony is especially illuminating. Twelve Franciscans were along, and a good number of younger sons of the nobility. They had brought insufficient food and supplies and were totally unprepared for the conditions they soon faced on the island. Almost as soon as they arrived a large number left to search for precious metals. After just over a week of grueling work, the food of most of these gold-seekers ran out, and the hungry miners returned to the city of Santo Domingo in search of elusive provisions. "They were tested in this fashion with the new land giving them fevers," Friar Bartolomé de Las Casas later remembered. They lacked food, medicines, and supplies, and they "began to die in such number that it was impossible for the priests to bury all. More than 1,000 of the 2,500 died, and 500 of them, with great affliction, hunger, and needs, remained ill."[82] In 1503 the first hospital in the Americas, named after San Nicolás, was founded in Santo Domingo for the cure of the poor, who were predominantly Spaniards.

Although the death rate for Europeans in the Americas during their first critical years of "seasoning" was quite high, it was nothing in comparison to the massive die-off of the natives. Bartolomé de las

82 Las Casas, *Historia de Indias*, 2:226.

Casas was an eyewitness to that disaster. The friar later sorrowfully commented on the rapid disappearance of the native population of the island during the administration of Governor Ovando. "The multitude of vecinos and peoples that there were on this island were being consumed, that according to the Admiral in a letter to the monarchs had been without number . . . and in the said eight years of that administration more than nine of ten parts perished. From here this drag-net passed to the island of San Juan [Puerto Rico] and to Jamaica, and afterwards to Cuba, and after that to Tierra Firme, and thus it spread and infected and devastated all this sphere."[83] The food shortages brought on by the poorly supplied massive attempts at colonization not only caused a heavy death rate for the unprepared Europeans, but the native Americans suffered too. The outsiders either forced the Indians to provide food or stole it directly from the fields or storage containers. Famine and disease were once again closely intertwined. Las Casas mentions "fevers" for the late 1502 to early 1503 period, but they are incompletely described, so diagnosis is risky.

THE FOURTH EXPEDITION

Columbus's ill-fated fourth voyage of discovery that set out three months after the Ovando fleet had left Andalusia also must have led to the introduction of disease, this time to the mainland of Tierra Firme. Four ships with a crew of 140 left Cádiz on 9 May 1502, stopping first on the coast of West Africa, where Columbus offered to assist the Portuguese, who were under siege at Arzila in Morocco. Because the siege had been lifted, the Spaniards remained only a day and then continued to the Canaries. There they loaded on water and provisions and sailed for the Indies on 29 May. Within twenty-one days they reached Martinique (15 June), where they secured fresh water and firewood. They sailed on to Dominica, Puerto Rico, and finally Santo Domingo, anchoring there on 29 June. Columbus intended to purchase a new ship, for one of his fleet was leaking badly, but Governor Ovando, worried about Columbus's intentions, ignored his inquiry. Columbus was concerned about a developing storm and requested permission to harbor, but the newly arrived governor refused his petition. Ovando was completing the outfitting of a large

83 Ibid., 2:257; and Frank Moya Pons, *Después de Colón; Trabajo, sociedad y política en la economía del oro* (Madrid: Alianza Editorial, 1987), pp. 29–52.

fleet of twenty-eight ships to send back to Spain; one of the passengers was the rebel Roldán. The Admiral warned Ovando about the weather; nonetheless the ships were dispatched. Columbus's intuition proved accurate, and a hurricane buffeted the fleet as they sailed in the Mona passage off eastern Hispaniola. All but three or four ships went down, hundreds perished, including Roldán and Francisco de Bobadilla. A large quantity of gold that was being sent back to Spain sank to the seabed.[84] Columbus's small fleet was scattered, but none of the ships foundered, and by 14 July they were able to depart Hispaniola, heading west.

The expedition reached the mainland off Honduras, encountering at Bonacca (now Belize) a native trade canoe, eight feet wide and as long as a Mediterranean galley, with twenty-five paddlers, a palm shelter amidships, and trade goods including swords, cotton shirts, clouts, sheets, copper axes, copper bells, roots, and grains. Such an excellent native trading vessel, one of many seaworthy crafts found in the Caribbean by the early Spanish, could have traveled easily anywhere in the Caribbean basin or along the Pacific coast, carrying products, people, and pathogens. Indeed, Columbus had mentioned in his log of the first voyage that on Cuba's northeast coast on 30 November 1492 they encountered a dugout canoe 95 palms long (about 65 feet) that was capable of carrying 150 people.[85]

The fleet sailed slowly southward, exploring the coastline along the way. In early November the explorers entered the harbor of Portobello, "well populated and surrounded by extensive country . . . full of houses."[86] Bartolomé and Columbus's son Ferdinand were members of the fleet. Many years later Ferdinand described events in his biography of the Admiral. When reading his long description of the isthmus region, of towns and people and cultivated fields, one cannot help but be struck by the lack of mention of disease that figures so prominently in Spanish accounts of the region two decades later. Yet in the rambling personal plea of Christopher Columbus to the monarchs dated Jamaica 7 July 1503, at a time when the fortunes of Columbus seem to be at their nadir, illness was mentioned. He mentioned his own sickness in his report of services to the Crown. He lamented the lack of rewards and the difficult position that he found himself in, shipwrecked as he was, without immediate hope of rescue. Along the

84 Floyd, *Columbus Dynasty*, p. 55.   85 Morison, *Journals of Columbus*, p. 107.
86 Ibid., p. 336.

coast, from what is today Honduras to Panama, he had suffered sickness. "I had become ill, and many times approached death."[87] At
another point, he related that he was "with strong fever, and so
fatigued that the only hope of escape was death."[88] And during a
terrible storm, one of an almost constant stream of torments that beset
the expedition, Columbus wrote, "I became so much fatigued that I
lost consciousness. It was there that I treated the sore [llaga] in the sea
water." Las Casas reports, "All this time the Admiral was suffering
from gout . . ." and "the men were ill too, sick and fatigued, and most
seasick."[89] Ferdinand also fell ill: "The pain of the son that I had there
tore at my soul, so much the more to see him at the tender age of 13,
in such lassitude and persisting in it so long."[90]

The fourth expedition of Columbus, as well as earlier ones, may
have led to the introduction of malaria to the American coasts, for
many of the first expeditionaries carried Vivax malaria, endemic in
Mediterranean Spain, in their blood. From mid-August 1502 until
April 1503, the men of Columbus coasted Mesoamerica. Mosquitoes
were so abundant that one section of the mainland came to be known
as the Mosquito Coast. One piece of evidence is to be found in the
condition of the man who would make possible the escape of Columbus from the shore of Jamaica. The explorers had reached the island of
Jamaica in May 1503. Two of the four worm-infested ships of the
original expedition had already been scuttled. One of the ships was
left on the mainland, and they had to give up a second on the voyage.
Inauspiciously, Columbus was forced to run aground their remaining
two worm-infested and badly leaking ships in the surf on the north
shore of Jamaica.[91] With the Admiral shipwrecked and ill on the
north coast of the island of Jamaica, Diego Méndez offered, with the
help of Indian oarsmen, to attempt to reach Hispaniola by canoe to
secure help. It was a difficult crossing between the islands; he suffered
terribly from heat and lack of water. By the time Méndez reached the
coast of Hispaniola, he was suffering from "a quartan ague caused by
all he had been through on land and sea."[92] Was this apparent fever
caused by sunstroke, insufficient water and food, or was Méndez suffering from a long-term illness he carried? The term used, quartan ague,
commonly described the principal symptoms of malaria. Davies argues

87 Cohen, Four Voyages, p. 286.   88 Ibid., p. 290.
89 Las Casas, Historia de Indias, 2:287.   90 Cohen, Four Voyages, p. 286.
91 Sauer, Early Spanish Main, pp. 121–36.   92 Cohen, Four Voyages, p. 365.

that Columbus, who became so ill at this point during the expedition, "probably had malaria, which would explain his delirium and ravings."[93] Fernández-Armesto also concludes that Columbus experienced malaria on the fourth voyage.[94] Actually, Columbus, Méndez, or anyone else on the fourth expedition could have been the European source of isthmanian malaria, the scourge that soon became such a threat to human settlement in the region. Any one of hundreds of Mediterranean Europeans suffering from quartan fevers could have inadvertently brought the malady to the Americas. López de Gómara reports that Hernán Cortés was unable to join the large Nicolás de Ovando fleet bound for Hispaniola in 1502 because he suffered a quartan fever in addition to an injury from an accidental fall from a crumbling wall while hurriedly leaving the bedroom of his lady. He did embark on his Atlantic venture in 1504.[95]

Nonetheless, the origin of New World malaria remains unresolved. In 1495 Michele de Cuneo wrote of the ubiquity of mosquitoes, the carriers of malaria, in the islands: "There are plenty of mosquitoes in those countries which are extremely annoying, and that is why the Indians anoint their bodies with those fruits which are red or black in color, and which are an antidote to their annoyance; but we could not find better remedy than stay in the water."[96] Fernández de Oviedo and other observers mentioned bothersome mosquitoes: "There are many mosquitoes, and very vexing, and of many types."[97] Several varieties of the *Anopheles* mosquito that could carry malaria existed in the Americas, waiting only for the introduction of the parasite into them via an infected Old World sailor.[98] Malaria was common in Mediterranean Europe in the late fifteenth century. If Diego Méndez did carry malaria, he survived to a ripe age, dying many years later in Spain, but then *Plasmodium vivax* (quartan malaria) can lie in the host for a lifetime, periodically debilitating the victim, but without killing.[99] The Amerindian rowers that accompanied Méndez from Jamaica to Hispaniola did not fare so well. They stopped on

93 Davies, *In Search of Columbus*, p. 245.
94 Fernández-Armesto, *Columbus*, p. 163.   95 López de Gómara, *Cortés*, p. 9.
96 Morison, *Journals of Columbus*, p. 220.
97 Gonzalo Fernández de Oviedo y Valdés, *Sumario de la natural historia de las Indias* (México: Fondo de Cultura Económica, 1950), pp. 188–89.
98 Frederick L. Dunn, "Malaria," in *Cambridge World History*, ed. Kiple, pp. 855–62.
99 Ibid., p. 856.

a small rocky island off the southwestern coast of Hispaniola to find drinking water. Only surface rainwater could be found in small depressions in the rock, and it was contaminated. "Some of the wretched Indians died there, and others incurred grave illnesses, in such fashion that few or none was fortunate enough to return to his homeland."[100]

The Spaniards who awaited rescue on the north shore of Jamaica soon faced difficulties of their own. Food brought from Tierra Firme quickly ran out. Columbus complained, "When the canoes had departed for Hispaniola the people left on board the vessels began to fall ill by reason of the hardship endured during the voyage and their change of diet; for no longer were they eating as in Castile, nor drank they any wine, nor could they get meat, save for a few hutias."[101] Columbus was so seized by arthritis (or perhaps gout) "that he could scarcely stir in his bunk."[102] Other men also fell sick. Securing ample food from the islanders was a major problem, as days became weeks, then months. Columbus's skillful manipulation of Jamaican natives, by forecasting an eclipse, seemingly empowered the Europeans with supernatural strength and helped to save them from Indian attack until they were rescued fourteen months after they were shipwrecked. Columbus's last return to Spain was difficult; much of the time he "could not rise from his bed from arthritis."[103] He reached the peninsula in November of 1504, and on 20 May 1506 he died in Valladolid, "much oppressed with his arthritis."[104]

TIERRA FIRME AND BEYOND (1504–1518)

Both nearby and more distant islands and even the mainland of the circum-Caribbean must have also been infected by Old World diseases by the end of the first quarter century following contact in 1492. Regions far to the north and the south, the fisheries of Newfoundland and the torrid lands of Brazilian dyewoods likewise were touched by potential carriers of Old World pathogens. Three principal types of economic activities quickly evolved. First, there was initial coastal reconnaissance. Second, there were the interior ventures with a fixed

100 Las Casas, *Historia de Indias*, 2:307.
101 Morison, *Journals of Columbus*, pp. 357–58.
102 Ibid., pp. 358–59.   103 Ibid., p. 369.
104 Sauer, *Early Spanish Main*, pp. 141, 155; and Morison, *Journals of Columbus*, pp. 369–70.

objective, such as the Balboa trek across the isthmus of Panama in 1512. Third, there were ventures that involved the continued return to areas of rich natural resources, such as the pearl fisheries off the coast of Tierra Firme, the fertile Newfoundland codfish banks in the north Atlantic, and the eastern coast of South America that was so rich in brazilwood. Some combination of types of ventures existed as well. The simple voyages of coastal discovery involved stops for taking on fresh water and whatever foods that could be secured by exchange (or theft if necessary), or occasional emergency repairs on ships that all too quickly fell victim to the ravages of hull worms. Many, if not most, of these expeditions resulted in direct contact between Europeans and native Americans. The Corte-Real brothers, Gaspar and Miguel, for example, sailing for the Portuguese, left a significant impact on the North American coast in 1500 and 1501. In the 1501 voyage they captured fifty-seven Indians of Newfoundland and carried them back to Portugal. The Indians had a "broken sword and a pair of silver earrings," an indication of possible face-to-face contact with members of the earlier John Cabot expedition or of other European voyagers. In 1508 or 1509, Sebastian Cabot sailed from England to Greenland and on northwestwardly to perhaps what became later Hudson Bay.[105]

Furthermore, several permanent settlements were established in Iberian New World territories. After the creation of Santo Domingo in 1496, a post was set up at Santa María de Belén on the north coast of Panama in 1502. In 1508 Diego de Nicuesa and Alonso de Ojeda received contracts to explore Veragua; the following year they succeeded in settling Urabá.[106] Nombre de Dios was established in 1510, and finally Panama City was founded on the Pacific side of the isthmus in 1519. The occupation of Cuba began in 1511. Santiago de Cuba was founded in 1514 and Havana in 1515. By that time, there were seven European settlements on the island. Ponce de León initiated the settlement of the island of San Juan (Puerto Rico) in 1508, but it had been touched by Europeans many times before, with earlier expeditions stopping for water, food, and supplies. The men of the second Columbus expedition of 1493 had stayed over between 18 and 21 November 1493, taking on provisions. The members of the 1499–

105 Russell Thornton, *American Indian Holocaust and Survival: A Population History since 1492* (Norman: University of Oklahoma Press, 1987), p. 14.
106 Floyd, *Columbus Dynasty*, pp. 95, 112.

1500 voyage of Diego de Lepe that coasted South America from the mouth of the Amazon to the Orinoco River visited Puerto Rico before beginning their return voyage to Seville. In 1504 or 1505, King Ferdinand had authorized Vicente Yáñez Pinzón to colonize Puerto Rico. He probably did come briefly and erect a stockade. In the same year, Juan de la Cosa received permission to explore Urabá, following up on the Bastidas expedition of three years earlier.[107]

Epidemic disease in Spanish cities and ports in the first decade of the sixteenth century is well documented. A severe drought and famine in 1505–6 contributed to conditions that were propitious for the propagation of disease. Mortality was so elevated that 1507 was called "the year of the great plague." Barcelona saw 3,500 deaths, Madrid 3,000; Valladolid 7,000; Avila 5,000, Zaragoza 12,000. About 100,000 victims fell to the malady in Andalusia, heartland of emigrants for the Indies venture.[108] Andrés Bernáldez, curate of the town of Los Palacios, describes the plight of his parishioners: "From the year 1502 there began to be in Castilla . . . much hunger and many illnesses of pestilential *modorra* and pestilence . . . until the present year of 1507, when they began in the month of January . . ., at the beginning of the year, in Jerez de la Frontera, and in Sanlúcar el Recio, and in Seville, and within all its jurisdiction, that ignited as a flame of fire."[109] Floyd links this epidemic sequence to events on the island of Hispaniola. Unless Andalusian harbormasters practiced quarantine for outbound ships, export of epidemic disease on board the fleets was likely. Floyd argues for the connection that "the Indian population had begun to decline especially in 1507–8, owing in all likelihood to the transmission to the Indies of the epidemic then raging in southern Spain."[110]

The total volume of possible contact between Amerindians and Europeans during this initial quarter century was substantial. In 1508 alone, forty-five ships sailed from Spain to Hispaniola, and, according

---

107 Ibid., p. 89; Sauer, *Early Spanish Main*, pp. 158–59.
108 Juan Ballesteros Rodríguez, *La peste en Córdoba* (Córdoba: Diputación Provincial, 1982), p. 42.
109 Andrés Bernáldez, *Memorias del reinado de los Reyes Católicos* (Madrid, 1962), p. 667. Bernard Vincent, "Las epidemias en Andalucía durante el siglo XVI," *Asclepio* 29(1977):351–58, found excellent information on this outbreak in city council deliberations and in correspondence of the Count of Tendilla.
110 Floyd, *Columbus Dynasty*, p. 95. He was unable to identify the disease (p. 243).

to the meticulous research of the Chaunus, between 1509 and 1515, 185 ships sailed to the Indies; 175 returned to the Old World during the same period.[111] The exploration of Florida likewise began early; Juan Ponce de León made his celebrated venture in 1513. In 1518 Hernández de Córdoba was killed in a skirmish with Indians along the Florida coast. In 1519 Alonzo Alvarez de Pineda laid claim to 300 leagues of the coast. In 1521 Ponce de León lost his life to Florida natives in his final attempt on the peninsula. Farther northward on the American mainland, in 1515 the Portuguese Estebán Gómez, acting for Spain, captured fifty-eight Indians in New England and transported them to Spain. He may have returned to the northeastern coast of the continent in 1524. In 1515 Lucas Vázquez de Ayllón raided and captured Indian slaves in what is now South Carolina; in 1526 he established a short-lived colony at Cape Fear.[112] More significantly, there must have been frequent unrecorded contacts along the east Florida coast following shipwrecks when fleets taking advantage of the currents on their return to Spain were caught in violent storms and cast upon the sandy beaches.

The exploration and settlement of the isthmus region between North and South America was of critical importance in future political events and especially in the dissemination of disease. Francisco Guerra argues that the swine flu that entered the Caribbean in 1493 reappeared in the isthmus district no later than 1517. If not swine flu, then some other illness was rampant on the isthmus of Panama shortly after the discovery of the "South Sea" by Vasco Núñez de Balboa in 1513.

There is clear evidence that in the 1514–17 period disease was introduced into the Darién district by the members of the Pedro Arias de Avila (often called Pedrarias) expedition. A long report about the ill-fated group was sent to Spain by Licentiate Zuazo. Approximately 1,500 men had been recruited in Seville, and "all or most of the men had been in Italy with the Gran Capitán." They left Sanlúcar de Barrameda aboard seventeen ships on 12 April 1514, and spent sixteen days on the island of Gomera provisioning and repairing ships.[113] The voyage to Dominica required only twenty-seven days. They stopped

---

111 Ibid., pp. 68, 255; Pierre and Huguette Chaunu, *Seville et l'Atlantique (1504–1650)*, 12 vols. (Paris: Colin, 1956–60), 2:20–23.
112 Thornton, *American Indian Holocaust*, p. 61.
113 Mártir, *Décadas*, p. 242; Licentiate Zuazo's report is provided in Sauer, *Early Spanish Main*, pp. 248–50.

there for water and firewood and then sailed on, reaching Santa Marta on the South American coast, where they faced hostile attack by the Indians. They continued to Cartagena and reached Darién around the middle or end of June 1514. Illness quickly struck. There was already a force of 450 of the Vasco Núñez expedition at Darién, and the 1,200 to 1,500 additional men of the Pedrarias group placed a severe strain on the ability of the settlers already there to feed them. The Pedrarias group included a large number of hidalgos and the leader's wife, Doña Isabel de Bobadilla. The settlement and surrounding district were swampy and wet; it was a place where "dense and sickly vapors rise, the men began to die and there died two-thirds of them, though dressed in silks and brocade." Andagoya, a participant, confirmed the account, writing that "the men began to sicken to such an extent that they were unable to care for each other and thus in one month seven hundred died of hunger and *modorra*." The historian and bureaucrat Gonzalo Fernández de Oviedo participated in the ill-fated venture and lamented that "more had died or left than remained in the country."[114] He too identified the malady as *modorra*.

There is no mention that either the previous Balboa party or the natives at the time had experienced severe illness, so it appears that the sickness was introduced from Europe. One must note that starvation coincided with the passage of the disease, for the leaders had not brought enough food supplies with the fleet to support the settlement for more than a few days. Las Casas reported that hidalgos dressed in silk could be found begging in the streets for food. "So many died daily that in one pit they dug, many were interred together, and at times if they excavated a grave for one of them they did not want to close it, because they knew for certain that within a few hours another might die to accompany him."[115] Even Pedrarias, in spite of better food rations, was stricken. From the Darién base Pedrarias sent his nephew, also named Pedrarias, to sail eastward 30 leagues with 200 men to explore the Cenú River, which was rumored to be rich in gold. They ascended the swift river with great difficulty. Most of the men were new and untried, and in addition they suffered the molestations of "the large number of mosquitoes that attacked them. . . . They began to fall ill and die." The nephew finally returned to Darién but not before losing half his men.[116]

114 Sauer, *Early Spanish Main*, pp. 249–50.
115 Las Casas, *Historia de Indias*, 3:38.   116 Ibid., 3:43.

Many have debated the nature of the illness called *modorra* that was so disastrous during the Pedrarias campaign and at other times and places during the sixteenth century. Rodrigo de Molina published in the city of Cádiz in 1554 a treatise on pestilence, in which he speaks of a sickness "called *modorra* by the common people."[117] Unfortunately Molina failed to describe its symptoms. Pérez Moreda suggests that an epidemic described as *modorilla* that swept Segovia in 1522 could have been bubonic plague.[118] Parry, on the other hand, suggests that *modorra* "may have been a deficiency disease" that afflicted travelers whose food on the voyage to the Indies had been inadequate. He argues that the supply of foodstuffs did not improve when the soldiers landed, for the settlers there were unable to produce the crops to feed such a large group.[119] But the Spanish term *modorra*, according to several sixteenth-century medical treatises, is fairly consistent, and the symptoms suggest a true epidemic sickness, not a deficiency disease. Influenza symptoms are similar to those described for those suffering with *modorra*. Influenza victims suffer lethargy for several days; their defenses are weakened, and they are prone to come down with more deadly ailments. Inadequate food, as contemporaries frequently mentioned, clearly exacerbated the problem.

Francisco López de Gómara perspectively describes the symptoms of *modorra* in his biography of Hernán Cortés. Licentiate Luis Ponce de León had been ordered (ca. 1526) to New Spain to conduct the residencia of Hernán Cortés. Licentiate Ponce de León attended mass at the Convent of San Francisco in Mexico City, and according to the biographer "retired to his lodgings suffering from a high fever, occasioned by the *modorra*. He took to his bed and was unconscious for several days, his fever and drowsiness increasing all the while. He died on the seventh day. Dr. [Cristóbal de] Ojeda, who attended him, treated him for *modorra* and swore it was the cause of death." Ponce de León had lost the power of speech the day he succumbed to the malady. "Of the hundred persons who had embarked with the Licenciado Ponce de León, most died at sea, or on the road within a few days

117 Sauer, *Early Spanish Main*, p. 250.
118 Vicente Pérez Moreda, *La crisis de mortalidad en la España interior (siglos XVI–XIX)* (Madrid: Siglo Veintiuno, 1980), p. 249. Plague may afflict simultaneously both human and some mammalian populations.
119 John H. Parry, "A Secular Sense of Responsibility," in *First Images of America: The Impact of the New World on the Old*, 2 vols., ed. by Fredi Chiappelli (Berkeley: University of California Press, 1976), 2:300.

of landing; of the Dominican friars, two. It was believed that a pestilence struck down and killed the others."[120] Ernesto Schafer described
the symptoms of the illness of Ponce de León to G. Sticker, professor
of the history of medicine at the University of Würzburg; his diagnosis
of the malady was epidemic meningitis.[121]

Past confusion over the exact nature of *modorra* might have been
cleared up by textual examination of the early seventeenth-century
lexicographer Covarrubias, who surely consulted contemporary medical treatises. Covarrubias describes *modorra* as "an illness that removes
the senses from man, much burdening [cargandole] the head." *Modorro*
can refer to "one who is with this [heavy, sleepy, drowsy] illness."
Another related meaning suggests that "sometimes it is said of the
person who is sluggish [*tardo*], silent [*callado*], and melancholic [*cabiz-
bajo*]." Covarrubias separately defines *modorilla* as "sickness of sheep."
Sticker's diagnosis of epidemic meningitis is certainly plausible, although other culprits remain as potential candidates. *Encephalitis lethargica* is one of the alternatives. Often coinciding with or following
influenza outbreaks, this ailment causes victims to display fever, lethargy, and disturbed eye movement. Other symptoms include "headache, tremor, weakness, depression, delirium, convulsions, the inability
to articulate ideas, coordinate movements, or to recognize the importance of sensory stimuli, as well as psychosis and stupor." Young adults
seem to be most frequently afflicted, and mortality in untreated modern cases is about 30 percent. Typhus is also a candidate.[122]

The Darién–Panama region was soon regarded by the Europeans as
a most unhealthy place, one to be avoided or to be rushed through as
quickly as possible. Fevers, probably malarial after the disease became
endemic, inflicted great damage to both permanent residents and a
large transient population. Pedro Mártir, basing his description on
eyewitness accounts, pointed out that Santa María de la Antigua was
inauspiciously located: "The situation of the place is morbific and
pestiferous, more pernicious than the climate of Cerena; everyone
becomes pallid as those who have jaundice (*ictericia*)." The sun, almost

---

120 López de Gómara, *Cortés*, p. 382. The translator Lesley B. Simpson incorrectly argued that *modorra* is a disease of sheep but that it is "defined too
vaguely for identification."
121 Ernesto Schafer, *El Consejo Real y Supremo de las Indias*, 2 vols. (Seville:
Imprenta M. Carmona, 1947), 2:4, 254–55.
122 R. T. Ravenholt, "Encephalitis Lethargica," in *Cambridge World History*, ed.
Kiple, pp. 708–10; Covarrubias, *Tesoro de la lengua*.

directly overhead, and the slow-moving polluted river, and the marshes contributed to the unhealthy scene. Many became ill: "The most noxious condition of the waters and of the air corrupted by the miasmatic emanations makes them ill," wrote the chronicler. Indeed, the description of the place by Mártir, who interviewed returnees, reminds one of the treatises describing conditions ideal for the plague. In contemporary belief, not only were vapors a cause for sickness, the soils and the general topographical features led to disease. "The place is also pestilential by the nature of the soil, marshy as it is, and surrounded by fetid lakes. Even more, the village is like a basin, where from the drops of water that flow through the hands of the slaves when they wash the floor of the house, at once toads are created, as I myself have seen in some places. And in summer those drops are converted into fleas."[123] It is interesting to remember that in the European mind the appearance of toads was a portent of a disastrous plague. The appearance of fleas in the Pedro Mártir account is intriguing, for they are associated directly with bubonic plague, even if at the time physicians did not recognize the scientific reasons. As a consequence of disease, and the flight of settlers to participate in the Peruvian venture, many towns were virtually abandoned. Oviedo, who was one of the original settlers of the district, and *regidor* of Darién in 1514 and Santa María de la Antigua in 1522, invested substantial resources. His two-story stone house in Santa María cost more than 1,500 castellanos to construct; it boasted a garden of sweet and sour oranges, lemons, and apples. Years later, when Oviedo completed his history, the place was a ghost town.[124] (See Table 1.2.)

GORJÓN'S TESTIMONY

Others, contemporaries of Bartolomé de las Casas, identified disease as one of the factors causing the rapid depopulation of the islands of the Caribbean. Around 1520, Hernando Gorjón, a *vecino* (resident with legal rights) of the small village of Azúa located on the south coast of Hispaniola, just to the west of Santo Domingo, wrote an informative though relatively unknown account of the early days of settlement. Gorjón reflected that he had come to the Indies with the fleet of

123 Mártir, *Décadas*, pp. 254–55.
124 Oviedo y Valdés, *Sumario de la natural historia* (México: Fondo de Cultura Económica, pp. 135, 146, 199.

Table 1.2. *Epidemic occurrences, circum-Caribbean, 1493–1525*

Year	Epidemic	Location
1493–8	Influenza, sickness	Hispaniola
1496	Sickness, jaundice	On voyage to Spain
1498	"Epidemic" syphilis (?)	Hispaniola
1500	Sickness, fevers	Hispaniola
1502	Illnesses general, fevers	Hispaniola
1507	Illnesses general	Caribbean to mainland
1514–17	Influenza (*modorra*)	Isthmus of Panama
1518–25	Smallpox pandemic	Caribbean to mainland

Governor Ovando in 1502. He recalled that when he first landed on the island, there had been many towns and people. These had gradually disappeared. He laid blame for the failure of the island's settlement on several factors: "Many Spaniards have gone, and the pestilence of smallpox, measles, and *romadizo* [Covarrubias states that *romadizo* is the same as *catarro*, or upper respiratory flu] and other illness, they [the Europeans] have given to the Indians."[125] As we have seen, another witness, Nikolaus Federmann, on the island from 1529–30 and 1531–32, reported that of 500,000 Indians on Hispaniola when the Spaniards first arrived, fewer than 20,000 remained when he wrote. For Federmann, the causes for decline were smallpox, warfare, and exploitation by the Spaniards. Gorjón's testimony is a decade earlier and is based on a much fuller experience with the islanders than Federmann's.

The epidemic of *romadizo* might refer to 1493–94, or 1502–7, or perhaps 1514, when serious illnesses assaulted the residents of Panama. Gorjón's mention of measles may be misleading; most historians date the initial measles pandemic from 1531. But the characteristic skin eruptions or rash provoked by measles resemble many other maladies, so eyewitnesses could have been confused. Hernando Gorjón's testimony indicates that several epidemics buffeted Hispaniola before 1520, thus demonstrating that the aboriginal Taino had not been swept away by a single watershed smallpox pandemic of 1518 but had

125 Rodríguez Demorizi, *Los Dominicos*, pp. 13–14; from *Colección de documentos inéditos*, 1:428.

suffered significant mortality earlier. It was not only the epidemic of influenza of 1493–94, identified by Francisco Guerra, but a series of other diseases that, working in combination, depopulated the island paradise so vividly described by Christopher Columbus, Michele de Cuneo, Bartolomé de las Casas, and other observers. At the end of the first quarter century after Old and New World contact, the Taino and their circum-Caribbean neighbors were approaching extinction.

CHAPTER TWO

The Deaths of Aztec Cuitláhuac and Inca Huayna Capac

THE FIRST NEW WORLD PANDEMICS

In the past year of 1518, smallpox, until now unknown by them, was ignited among them as flocks infected by contagious vapours.

Pedro Mártir

No one could move, not even turn their heads. One could not lie face down or on the back, or move from one side to another. When they did move, they screamed.

Native informant for Bernardino de Sahagún

The First Pandemic: Smallpox

Sickness and death came to the Americas with the second Columbus fleet in late 1493. In the first quarter century before the initial New World outbreak of smallpox in 1518, the worst killer of the Columbian exchange, the native populations of many of the islands of the Caribbean had already fallen sharply and most were nearing extinction. Nevertheless, the first smallpox epidemic was a watershed in the history of the peoples of the Caribbean and the mainlands beyond. The memory of that tragic event persisted long in the mind of the survivors, both the native Americans who suffered its debilitating scourge and the Europeans who witnessed their abundant labor force being annihilated.

The earliest documentary evidence for this devastating epidemic comes from the Jeronymite friars Luis de Figueroa and Alonso de Santo Domingo, writing from Hispaniola on 10 January 1519 to Charles V. The friars reported that the pestilence, which probably began in December 1518, had already taken the lives of almost one-third of the natives of the island and that at present it continued to rage unabated. "It has pleased Our Lord to bestow a pestilence of smallpox among the said Indians, and it does not cease. From it have died and continue to die to the present almost a third of the said Indians. And Your Highness must know that all that is possible has been done, and continues to be done, to cure them."[1] They lamented, betraying a less than Christian sentiment, that if the epidemic contin‑ ued at its current fury for two more months, it would be impossible to extract any gold from the island's mines in 1519. The friars reported further that the smallpox epidemic had spread to Puerto Rico: "We have been notified that already some Indians of the Island of San Juan have begun to die of the said smallpox."[2] A letter from the royal treasurer Haro directed to the king from Caparra (near modern San Juan) of Puerto Rico, on 21 January 1519, confirms the arrival of an epidemic on the nearby island. He reported that, although the natives were generally well treated, they died regularly, for they were "as weak in the body as they are in the faith."[3]

Other contemporaries bemoaned the terrible loss of life in the Caribbean. Pedro Mártir, who must have had access to the Jeronymite letters, and had prepared his text by 1520, reported that "in the past year of 1518, smallpox, until now unknown by them, was ignited among them as flocks infected by contagious vapours."[4] Bartolomé de las Casas, who wrote his description sometime after he returned to the island from Spain in 1520, provides a vivid account of the passage of the contagion. He must have queried both Indian and Spanish survi‑ vors for his history. He said "it was smallpox, and it was given to the pitiful Indians; it was carried by someone from Castile."[5] The Jeronym‑ ite friars in their correspondence of 10 January 1519 had failed to pinpoint the origin of infection, but they had indicated that its impact was less deadly for the Europeans. "From the said pestilence some few of our Spaniards have been stricken, but none have died; nonetheless

---

1 Salvador Brau, *La colonización del Puerto Rico* (San Juan: Instituto de Cultura Puertorriqueña, 1969), p. 315; and David Henige, "When Did Smallpox Reach the New World (and Why Does It Matter?)," in *Africans in Bondage: Studies in Slavery and the Slave Trade*, ed. Paul E. Lovejoy (Madison: University of Wiscon‑ sin Press, 1986), p. 17.

2 Brau, *Colonización*, p. 315.

3 T. S. Floyd, *The Columbus Dynasty in the Caribbean, 1492 to 1526* (Albuquerque: University of New Mexico Press, 1973), p. 190.

4 Pedro Mártir de Anglería, *Décadas del Nuevo Mundo* (Buenos Aires: Editorial Bajel, 1944), p. 346.

5 Bartolomé de las Casas, *Historia de Indias*, 3 vols. (México: Fondo de Cultura Económica, 1951), 3:270.

we are all fearful of the said smallpox, or another pestilence."[6] Las Casas concurs with the Jeronymites, noting that he had been told that few Spaniards were touched but that between one-third and one-half of the Indians had died.

Las Casas lamented the disappearance of the island Taino, writing that the epidemic left no more than 1,000 "of the immensity of peoples that this island held, and that we have seen with our own eyes." The Dominican friar also described the terribly quick death that came to those who, feverish, bathed in the rivers. The Spaniards, when they realized the devastation being caused by massive deaths, attempted to find an effective cure for the ill. Bartolomé de las Casas admonished that really "they should have begun it many years earlier." The Dominican suggested that the scarcity of adequate food, the native custom of nudity, the practice of sleeping on the ground, as well as excessive labor and lack of attention to health, all contributed to an elevated number of deaths.[7]

The passage of the smallpox epidemic on Hispaniola coincided with an Indian resettlement policy adopted by Judge Rodrigo de Figueroa. The native population of the island had already declined to the point at which, for the purposes of Christianization and proximity to a readily accessible labor supply, concentration of the reduced number of dispersed survivors seemed necessary to colonial officals and settlers. By the fall of 1518, Jeronymite friars, who oversaw the settlement policy, selected the sites of thirteen villages; five were inhabited by the spring of 1519. The smallpox epidemic began in the fall of 1518 and continued at least into January of the following year. But the death rate from smallpox was so great that it clearly reduced the population to the point that the forced resettlement of the remaining Tainos into villages was a farce.[8] It is not surprising that a native revolt broke out soon afterward. According to Las Casas, the uprising began near Xaraguá because an *encomendero* raped the wife of the cacique Ronquillo. On another level, Floyd believes the revolt may have been a reaction to the unpopular settlement policy. Clearly the futile explosion of rebellion was a bold act directed against alien control and the disaster that it brought to the Tainos. Unfortunately, the Tainos had been so quickly and thoroughly devastated that the effort to remove the foreigners had no chance for success.[9]

Disease also ravaged Iberian settlers, and recent immigrants soon

---

6 Brau, *Puerto Rico*, p. 315.   7 Las Casas, *Historia de Indias*, 3:270.
8 Floyd, *Columbus Dynasty*, p. 176.   9 Ibid., p. 192.

came to dread infection. This unease was justified, for Europeans, especially the newcomers, were regularly and quickly afflicted by illness. Judge Rodrigo de Figueroa wrote to Charles V from Santo Domingo on 6 July 1520 that fifteen days earlier a group of thirty-seven workers had arrived under the direction of Luis de Berrio. He complained that "they brought women, children and servants, and all fell ill; some are convalescing." On 16 September the same official wrote that "of the laborers who have come there so many have fallen ill that none remain, and some children and some women have died, and others become ill, in spite of the fact that they have been assisted." On 14 November 1520, in another report to the monarch, the official wrote "this year it has rained from May to now, and there have been an infinite number of sick."[10] Crosby speculated that the illness that swept the Caribbean at this time "was not an atypically pure epidemic. Smallpox seems to have been accompanied by respiratory ailments (*romadizo*), possibly measles, and other Indian killers."[11] We do note the concern voiced by the Jeronymites that other epidemics might be on their way. The likelihood of pneumonia cannot be discounted, for death by pneumonia was common among those suffering from smallpox, but Crosby's suggestion of the simultaneous presence of measles does not appear to be verifiable, at least on the basis of most extant evidence. Gorjón mentioned the possibility of measles too. One important difficulty is that, in one of the minor forms of smallpox, as medical specialist C. W. Dixon has indicated, the symptoms do resemble measles. Oviedo referred to the pandemic and its ravages in his history: "There occurred an epidemic of smallpox so virulent that it left Hispaniola, Puerto Rico, Jamaica, and Cuba desolated of Indians" or "with so few that it seemed a great judgment from heaven."[12]

THE AZTEC FIRST ENCOUNTER

The Aztecs called it *huey zahuatl*, or the big rash; at other times they referred to it as *totomonaliztli*. McCaa recently pointed out that the

10 Frank Moya Pons, *Después de Colón. Trabajo, sociedad y política en la economía del oro* (Madrid: Alianza Editorial, 1987), p. 171.
11 Alfred Crosby, *The Columbian Exchange: Biological and Cultural Consequences of 1492* (Westport, CT: Greenwood Press, 1972), p. 47.
12 C. W. Dixon, *Smallpox* (London: J. and A. Churchill, 1962); Gonzalo Fernández de Oviedo y Valdés, *Historia general y natural de las Indias, islas y Tierra Firme del mar océano*, 4 vols. (Madrid: Imprenta de la Real Academia de Historia, 1851–55), 1:105.

earliest mention of the central Mexican smallpox epidemic in European records is provided in a letter of the *oidor* (judge) of the Royal Audiencia of Santo Domingo, written to Charles V on 30 August 1520. In the missive, Licentiate Lucas Vázquez de Ayllón gave excellent details on the expedition of Pánfilo de Narváez, sent by the governor of Cuba to bring Hernán Cortés to justice. The fleet landed at Cozumel off the east coast of the Yucatán peninsula, finding there few natives left. Ayllón reported that the Indians had been stricken by disease brought by natives from Cuba. From Cozumel the flotilla continued in a northwesterly direction and finally landed at Cempoala, near Veracruz, probably on 4 March 1520. "Smallpox broke out almost immediately. Vázquez de Ayllón reports that great harm had been inflicted on those lands because smallpox had struck the Indians there. The report states unequivocally that smallpox was carried from Fernandina [Cuba] to the mainland by natives in the Narváez expedition."[13]

Smallpox entered the central valley of Mexico with the expedition sent from Cuba to deal with Hernán Cortés, precisely at the time that the contagion was raging through the Greater Antilles. Native informants who were questioned later by Friar Bernardino de Sahagún related that "while the Spaniards were still in Tlaxcala, a great plague of smallpox broke out among all the Indians."[14] Cortés had escaped recently from the great city during the chaotic and, for the Spaniards, disastrous retreat of the *Noche Triste* (the Sad Night) and was resting and recouping forces to begin a new assault on the Aztec capital. Indian witnesses reported that the disease began its course during the twelfth month in the festival of Teotlecco (10–29 September 1519). "The force of this pestilence lasted for sixty days. It killed innumerable people."[15] According to Cortés's biographer Francisco López de Gómara, "the Indians called this sickness *huitzahuatl*, meaning the 'great leprosy,' and later counted the years from it, as from some famous event."[16]

13 Robert McCaa, "Spanish and Nahuatl Views on Smallpox and Demographic Catastrophe in Mexico," *Journal of Interdisciplinary History* 25 (1995):403; the original report is that of Lucas Vázquez de Ayllón, "Relación que hizo el licenciado Lucas Vázquez de Ayllón, de sus diligencias para estorbar el rompimiento entre Cortés y Narváez," in *Cartas y relaciones de Hernán Cortés al Emperador Carlos V*, ed. Pascual de Gayangos (Paris, 1866), pp. 39, 42.

14 Bernardino de Sahagún, *Historia general de las cosas de Nueva España*, 8th ed. (México: Editorial Porrúa, 1992), pp. 744–45.

15 Ibid., p. 745.

16 Francisco López de Gómara, *Cortés, the Life of the Conqueror by His Secretary* (Berkeley: University of California Press, 1964), p. 205.

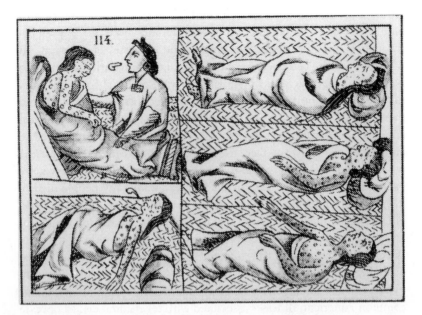

Figure 2.1. Mexicans ill with smallpox, from *Florentine Codex*.

Francisco López de Gómara provides another account of how the disease was transmitted from the islands of the Caribbean to Mexico's Gulf Coast. He wrote that "among the men of Narváez there was a Negro sick with the smallpox, and he infected the household in Cempoala where he was quartered; and it spread from one Indian to another, and they, being so numerous and eating and sleeping together, quickly infected the whole country."[17] Elsewhere the biographer of Cortés reports that "smallpox was introduced by a Negro of Pánfilo de Narváez."[18] Other contemporary sources mention introduction by an African slave. But several other sources fail to do so.[19] Whether or not he was the first in the party to sicken is unimportant, for it is clear that others, Cuban natives, in the Narváez camp carried the disease to the Mesoamerican shore. With the arrival of the pathogen on the coast of Veracruz, it was only a matter of time before the sickness spread.

According to the largely Tlaxcalan informants of Friar Sahagún, "It began in Cuatlán. When they finally took notice, it was already well developed. It went toward Chalco. And here its power diminished,

17 Ibid., pp. 204–205.   18 Ibid., p. 238.
19 McCaa, "Spanish and Nahuatl Views," p. 404.

although it did not completely end."[20] Beginning in the twelfth
month, after 10 September, it spread rapidly from 30 September
through 19 October, and, according to the witnesses of Sahagún, "It
was not until the celebrations of Panquetzaliztli [fifteenth month, 9–28
November] that the faces of our warriors were clean."[21] Contemporary
European descriptions of the symptoms are horrifying enough, but
there is added poignancy in the lamentations of those who were most
afflicted and voiced their agony: "Some were hit hard; it extended to
all parts of the body, the face, the head, the chest." It was not just the
pustules that were so painful, even quenching one's thirst caused
excruciating pain. "It was a dreadful illness, and many people died of
it. No one could walk; they could only lie stretched out on their beds.
No one could move, not even able to turn their heads. One could not
lie face down, or lie on the back, nor turn from one side to another.
When they did move, they screamed in pain."[22] Traditional Aztec
medicine failed to assist those stricken by the force of the infection.
Sweat baths, followed by cold ones, had been widely used to treat
common American illnesses associated with fevers. Francisco López de
Gómara described the results for Nahuatl peoples: "It was their custom
to bathe as a cure for all diseases, they bathed for the smallpox and
were struck down. They had the custom, or vice, of taking cold baths
after hot ones, so a man sick with the smallpox only escaped by a
miracle."[23]

In this case, as often happens when a terrible disease outbreak
devastates a population, so many fell infected that no one remained to
feed and nurse those who were recuperating. Countless people fled in
fear in order to avoid the contagion; parents left their children, hus-
bands their wives. "Many died from it, but many died only of hunger.
There were deaths from starvation, for they had no one left to care for
them. No one cared about anyone else."[24] The Spanish had witnessed
in the Old World the sad relationship between disease and starvation,
particularly during periodic outbreaks of the bubonic plague, which

20 Sahagún, *Historia general*, p. 791. Cuatlán is located in the jurisdiction of
     southeastern Hidalgo, under the administrative head of Acasuchitlan. It is due
     east of Pachuca and northeast of Cempoala, in the territory of Tulancingo; see
     Peter Gerhard, *A Guide to the Historical Geography of New Spain*, rev. ed.
     (Norman: University of Oklahoma Press, 1993), pp. 335–38.
21 Sahagún, *Historia general*, p. 792.   22 Ibid., p. 791.
23 López de Gómara, *Cortés*, pp. 204.
24 Sahagún, *Historia general*, p. 791.

frequently happened in the sixteenth century. López de Gómara describes the disaster in central Mexico: "And then came famine, not
because of a want of bread, but of meal, for the women do nothing but
grind maize between two stones and bake it. The women, then, fell
sick of the smallpox, bread failed, and many died of hunger."[25] Panic
and flight were all too common reactions to epidemic disease in
the sixteenth century. We now understand the mechanism by which
infection is passed on; they did not. Contact with the smallpox virus is
necessary for its spread. Contact could come directly from the material
in secretions in the nose and throat, could be carried in droplets in the
air, or could be passed by touch from the liquid in the pustules. The virus
could also persist ecapsulated in the scabs. When the virus entered the
victim's respiratory tract, the incubation was about eight to ten days before the manifestations: fever, malaise, then a generalized eruption on
about the third day of the onslaught, then the shift from papules to vesi-
cles, and finally pustules, if one lived that long.[26]

Variations in Aztec mortality were recognized by the Amerindian
informants of Sahagún. "Some people were hit with the pustules well
separated from one another; not many died from this. But many who
came down lost their good looks; they were deeply pitted and remained permanently scarred. Some lost their sight and became
blind."[27] Other symptoms are provided by a Nahuatl manuscript of
1528; it clearly describes the disease assault on Tenochtitlan while the
Spanish forces were in Tlaxcala following the *Noche Triste*. "Almost
the whole population suffered from wracking coughs and painful,
burning sores."[28] As a consequence of variations in mortality, it is
impossible to estimate accurately the overall loss of life in central
Mexico during this initial killer pandemic; nevertheless, it was appall-
ingly high. When the Spanish finally recaptured the Aztec capital,
"the streets were so filled with dead and sick people that our men
walked over nothing but bodies."[29]

The smallpox entered Mexico at a most propitious time for the

25 López de Gómara, *Cortés*, pp. 204–5.
26 Noble David Cook and W. George Lovell, "Unraveling the Web of Disease,"
   in *Secret Judgments of God: Old World Disease in Colonial Spanish America*,
   ed. Cook and Lovell (Norman: University of Oklahoma Press, 1992), pp. 217–
   18.
27 Sahagún, *Historia general*, p. 791.   28 Ibid., p. 814.
29 MaCaa, "Spanish and Nahuatl Views," pp. 428–30; Sahagún, *Historia general*,
   p. 847.

European invaders. Thrown out of the Aztec island capital of Tenochtitlan by the great native uprising, and losing a large number of troops
during the midnight escape that came to be known as the Noche
Triste, the outsiders were temporarily vulnerable. When Aztec ruler
Moctezuma died, his relative Cuitláhuac, the very capable lord of
Ixtapalapa, was chosen to replace him. To secure steadfast allies
against the Europeans, Cuitláhuac freed subjects from tribute contributions for a year. Furthermore, Cuitláhuac recognized that lances could
be used effectively against the foreign horse; this knowledge, coupled
with great numerical superiority, might have permitted some measure
of Aztec success against the outsiders. But his leadership was not
destined to last. Years later, Dominican Francisco de Aguilar, who
had been with Cortés during the conquest, remembered, "When the
Christians were exhausted from war, God saw fit to send the Indians
smallpox, and there was a great pestilence in the city."[30] The epidemic
lasted a little over two months in Tenochtitlan. By 13 August 1521
when Cortés retook the capital, according to López de Gómara, "the
enemy lost 100,000 men, or many more, according to others, but I am
not including those who died of hunger and the pestilence. . . . They
[the defenders] slept among the dead and lived in a perpetual stench,
for which reasons they sickened or were struck down by the pestilence,
in which an infinite number died."[31] Cortés himself, in a letter to the
emperor on 15 May 1522, linked the central Mexican epidemic and
that of the Antilles. He wrote that many of the native leaders had
died as a consequence of the "smallpox distemper which also enve-
loped those of these lands like those of the islands."[32]

One of those who died was the perceptive and capable Aztec ruler
Cuitláhuac.[33] (See Figure 2.2.) Fernando de Alva Ixtlilxóchitli wrote
that "Cuitlahuatzin did not rule more than forty days, because he died
of smallpox brought by a Black."[34] James Lockhart's translation of the
event in the native source Anales de Tenochtitlan (the Codex Aubin)
provides poignant testimony on the devastating event. "The tenth
ruler was installed in Ochpaniztli, Cuitlahuatzin. He ruled for only
eighty days; he died at the end of Quecholli [probably late November
or early December of 1520] of the pustules, when the Christians had

30 Crosby, Columbian Exchange, p. 48. My emphasis.
31 López de Gómara, Cortés, p. 293.
32 Hernando Cortés, Cartas de relación (México: Editorial Porrúa, 1971), p.
    105.
33 López de Gómara, Cortés, p. 239.   34 Sahagún, Historia general, p. 828.

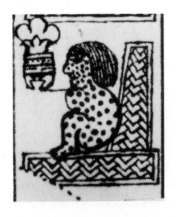

Figure 2.2. Depiction of one of the first (1520) Mexican smallpox victims, perhaps one of Cuitláhuac, from *Codex en Cruz*.

gone to Tlaxcala."[35] Pedro Mártir reported that he had ruled only four months, and "had died of smallpox and had been succeeded by his sister's son, Catamazin [Cuauhtémoc]."[36] In the *Crónica Mexicayotl* (written about 1609), we note that the ruler's son Axayacatzin was also killed by smallpox.[37]

The initial smallpox pandemic was disastrous for the Aztecs. McNeill's measured evaluation of its impact is appropriate; the smallpox had "paralyzed effective action, the Aztecs lapsed into a stunned inactivity."[38] Amerindian inaction gave the outsiders the edge; the foreigners conquered and remained. McCaa concluded that the native elite was devastated and that "the military significance of the pestilence was enormous."[39] Native accounts of the Spanish conquest of Mexico stress the fact that the terrible epidemic was more memorable than military conquest and death by the sword.[40] Spanish success in

35 James Lockhart, *We People Here: Nahuatl Accounts of the Conquest of Mexico* (Berkeley: University of California Press, 1993), p. 279.

36 MaCaa, "Spanish and Nahuatl Views," p. 408.   37 Ibid., p. 408.

38 William H. McNeill, *Plagues and Peoples* (Garden City, NY: Anchor Doubleday, 1976), p. 183.

39 McCaa, "Spanish and Nahuatl Views," p. 411.

40 Francis J. Brooks, "Revising the Conquest of Mexico: Smallpox, Sources, and Populations," *Journal of Interdisciplinary History* 24(1993):29, argued that smallpox had no impact on conquest and rejected demographic collapse outright. McCaa, "Spanish and Nahuatl Views," p. 398, rejected the revisionists, writing that there are new and "overlooked sources, misread texts, flawed reasoning, and false analogies." See also Henry F. Dobyns, "Disease Transfer at Contact," *Annual Review of Anthropology* 22 (1993):273–91, for a brief survey of the debates over disease.

taking and holding the Aztec heartland was linked, as Diego Muñoz Camargo wrote in the sixteenth century, to sickness. The War of Mexico had come to an abrupt ending, "because the illness that had recently hit them had left them so weak and sick."[41]

MAYA TRAGEDY

Smallpox came to the Yucatán peninsula at roughly the same time that it reached the Gulf Coast of Mexico. Friar Diego de Landa said that sometime near the end of the second decade of the century "there came a great pestilence, with great pustules that rotted the body, fetid in odor, and so that the members fell in pieces within four or five days." Actually the exact date is not clear, for Landa was not a direct witness and referred to the illness that passed "more than fifty years" before. If he wrote his description in 1566, the sickness would have taken place in 1516 or earlier.[42] Although the date Diego de Landa supplies for the Yucatán is imprecise, we do have a more precise view of the time at which smallpox entered the lands of the nearby Guatemalan Maya. The compilers of the *Annals of the Cakchiquels* recorded that "a great and mortal epidemic" swept into the area five years prior to the campaign of Pedro de Alvarado; that would have placed the epidemic's appearance in 1519. The description of symptoms is excellent, although translations of the Maya text have varied. Recinos and Goetz rendered the account as: "They became ill of a cough, they suffered from nosebleed and illnesses of the bladder."[43] Brinton earlier translated the text as: "First there was a cough, then the blood was corrupted, and the urine became yellow."[44] In Guatemala 1519 came to be known as the year in which "the plague raged." The following two years, 1520 and 1521, were known as the time when "the plague spread."[45] The dates of inception of the smallpox pandemic in central Mexico and the epidemic of Guatemala are close. If the original site of infection was Cempoala on Mexico's southern

41 McCaa, "Spanish and Nahuatl Views," pp. 425–26.

42 Crosby, *Columbian Exchange,* pp. 47–48; and Diego de Landa, *Yucatán before and after the Conquest* (New York: Dover, 1978), p. 19.

43 Adrián Recinos and Delia Goetz, eds., *The Annals of the Cakchiquels* (Norman: University of Oklahoma Press, 1953), pp. 115–16.

44 Daniel G. Brinton, ed., *The Annals of the Cakchiquels* (Philadelphia: Library of Aboriginal American Literature, 1885), p. 171.

45 W. George Lovell, "Disease and Depopulation in Early Colonial Guatemala," in *Secret Judgments,* eds. Cook and Lovell, p. 67.

Gulf Coast, then the chronological proximity is not difficult to explain.

It is important to note that pustules, mentioned by Diego de Landa in his account, and the most prominent characteristic of smallpox, are not included in the Cakchiquel text. This lapse has led to prolonged debate over correct identification of the Maya epidemic; some argue that it was probably an extension of the smallpox pandemic from central Mexico, whereas other specialists have suggested that it was more likely measles or another disease – influenza, exanthematic typhus, even pulmonary plague. Other Guatemalan sources that refer to this period are inconclusive. Many years later (1585) in a geographical description of San Bartolomé, prepared under orders of King Philip II, local informants reported that "before the Spaniards arrived in this land there was an incurable outbreak of smallpox." Some scholars have correlated this with the initial Mexican pandemic, but direct evidence of the date is inconclusive. George Lovell, who has studied carefully the Guatemalan episode, concludes that "the balance of commentary thus may favor smallpox, but not unanimously so. What seems worthy of observation is that medical doctors who analyze the native text are more inclined to diagnose measles than smallpox."[46]

The Maya record may be read in a variety of ways; Maya description of alien disease is garbled. Part of the reason is that individual symptoms even during the same epidemic varied, and the manifestations were similar yet at the same time dissimilar to diseases the Maya had experienced before the arrival of the outsiders. The wide range of possible symptoms of smallpox has already received attention. Furthermore, the great smallpox pandemic was followed in less than a decade by an almost equally devastating epidemic of a disease with not totally dissimilar symptoms. This second epidemic was probably measles. Perhaps there also occurred a bout of *landres*, or the plague. The primary source, the *Annals of the Cakchiquels*, was prepared long after the original events had taken place. It is likely that a blurring took place in the popular mind of the Amerindians about both symptoms and exact chronology. Such blurring is found to be true for two of the mestizo and native American accounts of the death of Inca ruler Huayna Capac in the Andean region of South America.

It is not surprising that the first smallpox pandemic that swept much of the Americas extracted such a heavy toll in human lives. Although levels of case mortality vary widely, as Dixon and other

46 Lovell, "Disease in Early Colonial Guatemala," p. 66.

specialists have demonstrated, ranging from a low of 10 percent to a high of almost 100 percent with fulminating smallpox, the critical factor is morbidity. The entire aboriginal population of America was at risk in the era of initial contact. No one had experienced smallpox, or measles, or any other alien infection. The Americas in that sense was a virgin land. Furthermore, when established in epidemic form, smallpox can spread rapidly, for it is transmitted by aerosols in addition to contact with the virus on infected objects such as clothing. Furthermore, as native and European testimony suggests, when almost everyone is stricken, there is no one left to feed or nurse the infected back to health. The disaster is complete. (See Map 2.1.)

In the Old World, in isolated regions where smallpox did not reach the population for two or three generations, the level of mortality was equally high. Documentation is sparse, but Dixon has pointed out that in South Africa and Iceland, where virtually virgin conditions existed, community mortality was about 35.36 percent.[47] Even with generations of exposure to smallpox, death rates remained high until vaccination cracked the cycle. Early in the eighteenth century smallpox was the cause of 10 to 15 percent of the deaths in several countries. Deaths of children from smallpox were numerous. Flinn points out that "80 percent of those deaths were children under ten, 70 percent of children under two."[48] Mercer points to community case fatalities of smallpox in nineteenth-century Verona at 46.70 percent, Milan at 38.50, and Bohemia at 29.80. For the Pueblo Indians in the same century it was 74 percent, and for Hawaii, 77.70.[49]

TAWANTINSUYU

Southward in the great Andean cordillera that stretches along the entire western coast of South America, the heartland of the great Inca empire, the first great smallpox pandemic ravaged Amerindian peoples. As in the example of Aztec Mexico, where the ruler Cuitláhuac succumbed to the foreign infection, the Inca ruler Huayna Capac fell victim to a hideous alien disease. Knowledge of the demise of the

---

47 Dixon, *Smallpox*, pp. 207–8.
48 Michael W. Flinn, *The European Demographic System, 1500–1820* (Baltimore: Johns Hopkins University Press, 1981), p. 63.
49 A. J. Mercer, "Smallpox and Epidemiological-Demographic Change in Europe: The Role of Vaccination," *Population Studies* 39(1985):302; and Thomas M. Whitmore, *Disease and Death in Early Colonial Mexico. Simulating Amerindian Depopulation* (Boulder, CO: Westview Press, 1992), p. 56.

leader of the land of the four quarters, Tawantinsuyu, comes secondhand in the form of oral history, as recorded by European observers a
few years after the actual event. The history of Andean America was
written primarily by the early Europeans or by Hispanicized mestizos,
not by the native Andeans. In contrast to the Mesoamerindians, who
had knowledge of writing, the Andean Americans did not. They did
make records and manipulated numerical quantities with great facility
on knotted-string mnemonic devices they called *quipus*. Chronologies
of dynasties and conquered peoples could have been recorded, but the
quipucamayo, as the person who kept the records was called, was
necessary to translate, to give meaning to, the knots in the colored
strings. Throughout the sixteenth century, in spite of the introduction
of the European alphabet in the Andean world, quipucamayos continued to record statistical data on tributaries, families, and tribute goods.

The first Europeans to write about the Andean world were, as
Christopher Columbus had been in the Caribbean, less interested in
history than in the richness of the land and its peoples. Accounts of
Pizarro's first expeditions reflect these concerns, for they were issues
that were paramount if new investors were to be convinced to support
continued expeditions to the south. The earliest reports did not mention Huayna Capac at all, only the current ruler Atahualpa, or his
half-brother Huascar, or local lords. The investment in the Peru venture did bring vast treasures to the bearded, light-skinned foreigners
(who were often called Viracocha) when they captured Huayna Capac's son Atahualpa and collected his ransom at Cajamarca in 1533.
The Spanish finally began to be interested in Inca history in the early
1540s. Their own position now seemed at last secure following the
defeat of the great native uprising of Manco Capac in 1537, and they
needed a thorough understanding of the peculiar history of the land
and its peoples in order to establish a stable colonial system. They also
needed to be able to distinguish legitimate from illegitimate claims of
members of the native elite, particularly the descendants of the Inca
lineage who were in theory exempt from tribute.[50]

50 James Lockhart, *Men of Cajamarca: A Social and Biographical Study of the First
   Conquerors of Peru* (Austin: University of Texas Press, 1972); Steve J. Stern,
   Peru's Indian Peoples and the Challenge of Spanish Conquest: Huamanga to 1640
   (Madison: University of Wisconsin Press, 1982); Noble David Cook, *Demo-
   graphic Collapse: Indian Peru, 1520–1620* (Cambridge: Cambridge University
   Press, 1981); Karen Spalding, *Huarochirí: An Andean Society under Inca and
   Spanish Rule* (Stanford: Stanford University Press, 1984); John Hemming, *The
   Conquest of the Incas* (London: Sphere Books, 1972).

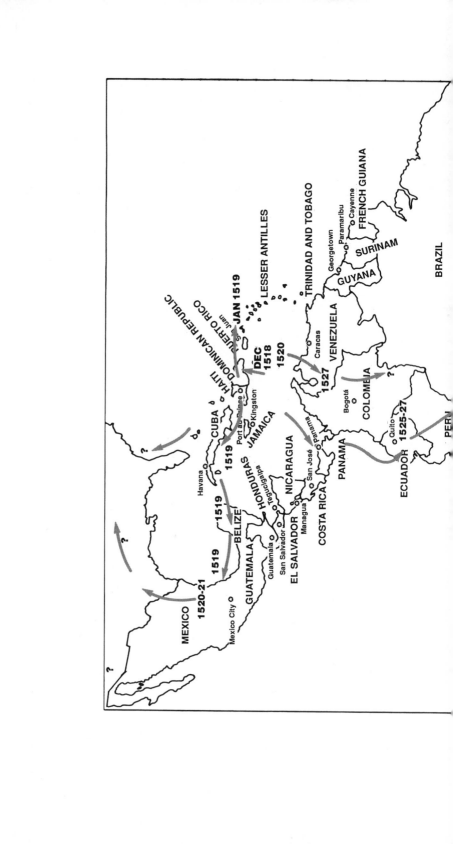

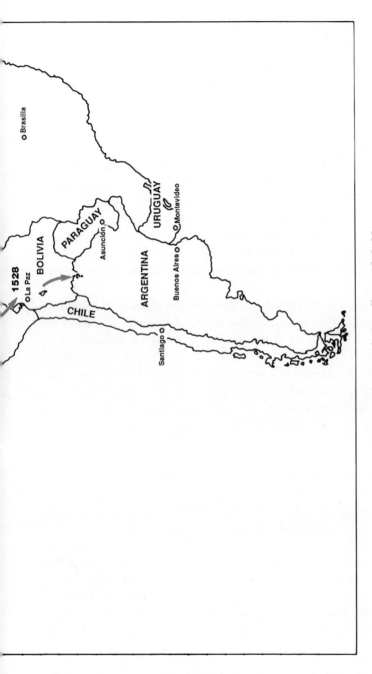

Map 2.1. The spread of smallpox, 1518–28.

Unfortunately the civil wars of the conquerors intervened, and it would not be until at the beginning of the next decade, the 1550s, that the Spaniards could turn to a serious search for the nature of the past of Tawantinsuyu. Two principal early figures in this search were Pedro de Cieza de León (1550, 1553) and Juan de Betanzos (1551).[51] Both had been fighters in the campaigns and were largely self-taught historians. Especially informative is the second part of the account of Betanzos, lost for so long in a private archive and not published in complete form until 1987. Betanzos probably entered the Caribbean in 1523 and traveled to Peru shortly after 1539. Juan de Betanzos came to know the Inca past well, much better than most Europeans did, for he married Inca princess (ñusta) Cuxirimay Ocllo, baptized Angelina. She had been Francisco Pizarro's concubine and had close contacts with members of the Inca royal lineage in Cuzco. Betanzos questioned his wife's relatives at length and prepared a Quechua dictionary and grammar.

Juan de Betanzos reported that after the conquest of the province of Yaguarcoche, Inca Huayna Capac returned to Quito and was there six years. At the end of that time, "he came down with an illness which deprived him of his senses and understanding, and gave him a sarna [cutaneous disease] and lepra [leprosy] that made him very debilitated, and the lords finding him in such state entered."[52] The native leadership questioned the ruler about succession; the Inca at first replied that his one-month-old son Ninancuyochi, who lived in the province of Cañares, should be the lord Inca. On subsequent days elders returned to the issue of succession; Huayna Capac named Atahualpa, and later Huascar. Four days later Huayna Capac succumbed to the malady. At this point the messengers who had gone to the infant originally named heir by Huayna Capac returned with news that "he had died of the same illness of lepra as his father."

Accurate dating of the event is difficult. Betanzos relates that during the Inca ruler's last days, the caciques of Tumbez approached him with news that the outsiders had arrived. According to Betanzos's description, this was when Francisco Pizarro first arrived at Tumbez with only fifteen to twenty men. They had gone as far as Paitá, and then Pizarro had returned to Spain for authorization from the

51 Franklin Pease G. Y., *Las crónicas y los Andes* (México: Fondo de Cultura Económica, 1995), pp. 191–243.
52 Juan de Betanzos, *Suma y narración de los Incas* (Madrid: Atlas, 1987), p. 200.

king to continue exploration and conquest. This account would place the Inca ruler's death sometime during the second Pizarro expedition, 1526–28.[53] In accordance with native tradition, the corpse of Huayna Capac was opened, the viscera removed, and the body was prepared and cured in the open air. After proper preparation, it was dressed in precious clothing and placed on a rich litter decorated with feathers and gold. The dead ruler was carried in state to Cuzco, accompanied by local lords and the mother and daughter of Huascar. The transfer of the corpse of Huayna Capac to the imperial capital, in keeping with the Inca tradition of veneration of the mummies of the ancestors, surely continued the inexorable spread of the epidemic, as all highland peoples from the Quito district to Cuzco came into contact with the ruler.

The smallpox virus, encapsulated in the scabs, is remarkably resistant to damage and can remain viable for weeks and even longer. Use of the words *sarna* or *lepra* by Betanzos to identify the illness simply indicates symptoms of severe skin rash and inflammations. These words had directly translatable equivalents in Quechua, the general language of the Incas found in the 1586 dictionary of Antonio Ricardo: *sarna* is "caracha" and *lepra* is "caracha llecte" (grime or filth). It is instructive to note that Ricardo defines both *sarampión* (measles) and *viruelas* (smallpox) as "muru oncoy" in Quechua. The definition of "muru" is seed, and here one should think of the seed of the large-kerneled Andean corn, which almost perfectly describes the seedlike rash. Oncoy simply translates as malady, or illness.[54]

Pedro de Cieza de León's account parallels that of Betanzos. Cieza also came to the Indies as a young man, involved first in the conquest and settlement of New Granada. He planned to compose a multivolume history of the Andes, beginning with flora and fauna, moving to the origins of the Incas, then detailing their discovery and conquest by the Europeans, and at last tracing their civil wars. He collected extensive notes and took them everywhere he traveled, writing in the mid-1540s. At the end of the Peruvian civil wars, he was befriended by president of the *audiencia* Pedro de la Gasca and secured authorization to interview both Spanish officials and remaining members of the Inca quipucamayos. The principal outlines of Cieza's description of the death of Huayna Capac are similar to those of Betanzos, whom he may

53 Ibid., pp. 200–201.
54 Antonio Ricardo, *Vocabulario y phrasis en la lengua general de los indios del Perú, llamada quichua* (Lima: San Marcos, 1951); the first edition was published in Lima, 1586.

have met. While the Inca ruler was in Quito, after the conquest of the
north, "a great pestilence of smallpox came, so contagious that more
than two hundred thousand souls passed away in all the surrounding
districts."[55] The chronicler reported that nowhere could one escape
the sickness. Huayna Capac felt that he had become infected and
ordered that sacrifices be performed throughout the realm for his
health. Cieza notes that there was divergence of opinion among his
informants. Some said that the Inca ruler divided the realm between
Huascar and Atahualpa, but others disagreed with the account of the
division. After the death of Huayna Capac, his *huaca* (Quechua word
referring to any spiritual force that could be represented by a physical
object) was carried with much lamentation from Quito to Cuzco.
There 4,000 women and servants in Cuzco were sacrificed to join the
ruler on his journey, a secondary cause of mortality arising from the
appearance of the pandemic.

Three principal accounts from the early 1570s and 1580s detailing
an epidemic cause of death of Inca Huayna Capac are those of Spaniard conquistador–settler Pedro Pizarro, soldier and bureaucrat Pedro
Sarmiento de Gamboa, and the cleric Miguel Cabello Balboa. All
accounts are based on a mixture of observation and secondhand information and clearly involve distillation of evolving native tradition.
Pedro Pizarro's history, completed about 1571, is the passionate account of a participant. In his version the Inca ruler had just conquered
Quito and to celebrate his victory was engaged in construction of a
fort, as was customary when the Incas subjugated a province. While
they were building it, there appeared among them "a sickness of
smallpox, never seen among them before, which killed many Indians."
Pizarro recollected that Huayna Capac was "at the time fasting, as
customary, remaining alone neither taking a woman, nor eating salt,
aji, nor drinking chicha . . . and three Indians never seen before
entered, very small like dwarfs. They approached the Inca, saying they
had come to call on him." As he experienced this vision he called his
advisers, and as they entered, the three dwarfs disappeared. No one
had seen them but Huayna Capac. The Inca asked his advisers, "For
what reason have these dwarfs come to call on me?" And they responded, "We have not seen them." Then Huayna Capac said: " 'I
must die,' and then he fell ill with smallpox." While he was ill,

55 Pedro de Cieza de León, *Señorio de los Incas* (Lima: Universidad Católica del
   Perú, 1984), pp. 219–20.

messengers (*chasquis*) were sent to Pachacamac to ask the oracle what could be done to secure the health of Huayna Capac. The witchdoctors spoke with the demon through the idol, and the demon replied that they should take the Inca out into the sunshine. Then he would be healed. But in so doing the opposite occurred, for by being placed in the sun Huayna Capac died.[56]

A second account written in the 1570s is that of Pedro Sarmiento de Gamboa, who entered Peru about 1557, after a long administrative career that had taken him from the wars in France in the 1550s to Mexico. Associated in Peru with Viceroy Francisco de Toledo, he was in charge of the collection of material intended to become the "official" history of the Incas. In Cuzco Sarmiento had the opportunity to interview closely a group of surviving quipucamayos. Unfortunately Sarmiento de Gamboa's report was a partisan one. Viceroy Toledo was collecting information to justify Spanish conquest and rule in the Andes, and part of that information was manipulated to prove that Inca rulers had been usurpers and unjust. Sarmiento was therefore especially interested in the origin of the Inca dynasty and the question of legitimate succession. In spite of the political purpose of Sarmiento de Gamboa's account, his story is remarkably similar in its basic outline to those of Betanzos and Cieza de León. Sarmiento places the date of the death of Huayna Capac at the end of 1524, during the nativity period in the Christian calendar.

While he was in the north, at the time of the conquest of the Huancavilcas, the Inca learned that there was in Cuzco "a great pestilence, from which his governors Apu Hilaquita, his uncle, and Auqui Tupac Inca, his brother, and his sister Mama Cuca, with many other of his relatives, died." When the Inca arrived in Quito, "he came down with an illness of fevers, although others say that it was of smallpox and measles. As a consequence, for he began to feel that he was going to die, he called the *orejones*, his relatives, who asked him whom he had chosen as his successor. He responded that it was his son Ninan Cuyoche and that if fortune gave a good sign, his son would succeed him well. And if not, it would be given to his son Huascar."[57] The sacrifices were made, Cusi Tupac Yupanqui, chief majordomo of the sun cult officiating. A camelidae was sacrificed, the

56 Pedro Pizarro, *Relación del descubrimiento y conquista del Perú* (Lima: Universidad Católica del Perú, 1978), pp. 48–49.

57 Pedro Sarmiento de Gamboa, *Historia de los Incas* (Madrid: Ediciones Polifemo, 1988), p. 148.

lungs removed, the veins examined. Neither omen was favorable to Ninan or to Huascar. They turned back to ask Huayna Capac to name another, but they found him already dead. Cusi Tupac Yupanqui said to go and notify Ninan that he had been chosen, "But when they arrived at Tumi-pampa [sic], they found that Ninan Cuyoche was dead of the pestilence of smallpox."[58] Sarmiento de Gamboa is the first to introduce the idea that the great Andean pandemic originated in the Cuzco district. Furthermore, although the chronicler seems confused as to the cause of Huayna Capac's death, mentioning alternatively fevers, smallpox, and measles, he reports that Ninan Cuyoche was mortally stricken by smallpox, with the implication that the same malady had killed Huayna Capac.

Miguel Cabello Balboa's history is especially valuable, for he knew the north coastal peoples better than most other early Spanish observers. He was probably born in Archidona in Malaga. He fought in the wars against the French, later becoming first an ecclesiastic and then finally a missionary. Cabello Balboa reached the Americas about 1566 and took holy orders in 1571. He traveled extensively through New Granada and Quito and joined in several *entradas* into the interior. He prepared an excellent geographical and ethnological account of the province of Esmeraldas on Quito's coast. He often served as chaplain and began collecting documents for his history in 1576. He had learned Quechua and interviewed quipucamayos during his inquiries. Cabello Balboa reports that after Huayna Capac completed conquests in the north, he paused in Tumibamba. He continued to the coast and reached the island of Puná, where he may have first been notified of the arrival of the *Viracocha* – the European. At Puná, Huayna Capac also "received very sad news from Cuzco, from where they informed him that there was an incurable and general pestilence that had taken his brother Auqui Topa Inca and his uncle Apo Illaquita, whom he had left as governors when he left Cuzco, and his sister Mama Toca, and other principal lords of his lineage."[59] Profoundly saddened by the news, Huayna Capac continued toward Tumibamba. He passed the Guayaquil River and took a little-frequented route through Mulluturu. From Tumibamba, "feeling indisposed and in ill health, he continued to Quito with the greatest and best part of the army, and arriving there

58 Ibid., p. 149.
59 Miguel Cabello de Balboa, *Miscelánea antártica* (Lima: San Marcos, 1951), p. 393.

his malady worsened, and turned into deadly fevers. Feeling himself near death, he made his testament according to their custom."[60] Cabello Balboa gives the date of the ruler's death as "according to our count, in the year 1525." His will, composed on quipus in the presence of many witnesses, named his much loved son "Ninancuyuchic, who at this very time was ill with fevers, from which in a few days he died."[61] As does Sarmiento de Gamboa, Cabello Balboa reports that the epidemic's force was first felt in Cuzco; otherwise, his account parallels those of others. Amidst great lamentation, Huayna Capac's body was embalmed and solemnly carried to Cuzco.

The accounts of the death of Huayna Capac come from various types of witnesses. (See Figure 2.3.) Although flawed, they provide the raw evidence for a series of generalizations. Clearly Huayna Capac became ill; most likely he was infected by the smallpox virus and succumbed to the disease between late 1524 and 1528, coinciding with European exploration southward along the Pacific Coast but several years before the outsiders entered the Andean highlands. There is much debate over the exact date of his demise. Sarmiento de Gamboa, who closely consulted surviving quipucamayos, stated that "Huayna Capac died in the year of fifteen twenty-four of the nativity of Our Lord Jesus Christ."[62] Many of Huayna Capac's compatriots, including close family members, died from the same illness. Most important for the foreign invaders of Tawantinsuyu, the Inca's death led directly to fratricidal strife between two brothers, Atahualpa and Huascar. This civil war was bloody and ruthless. Furthermore, ethnic entities that had been recently integrated into the Inca polity were only lukewarm in their loyalty to the Inca regime. Weakened by epidemic disease, civil war, and internal dissension, the native peoples of the Andean highlands fell easy prey to European encroachments. Superior technology is only part of the equation for the success of the Spanish in Peru, just as it is only one element in the explanation of the ease of conquest of Mesoamerica.

The death of Huayna Capac provides a vivid illustration of what

---

60 Ibid.   61 Ibid., p. 394.
62 Sarmiento de Gamboa, *Historia*, p. 149. David Henige, "Counting the Encounter: The Pernicious Appeal of Verisimilitude," *Colonial Latin American Historical Review* 2(1993):325–61, argues that all accounts are retrospective and therefore suspect. This is correct, but the evidence provided to the Spaniards in the Inca heartland indicates that there was serious illness before the arrival of the Europeans and that many, including the Inca ruler, died.

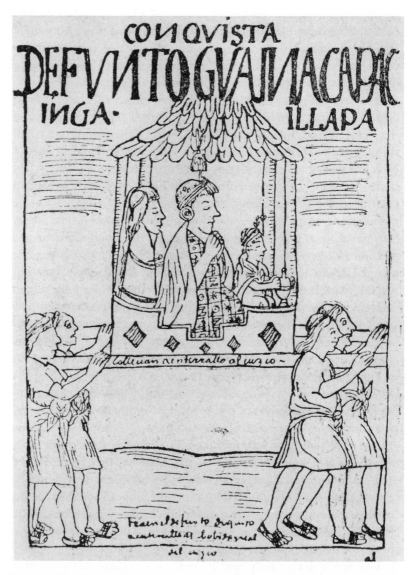

Figure 2.3. Huayna Capac's mummy bundle, sent to Cuzco, from Felipe Guaman Poma de Ayala, *Nueva corónica y buen gobierno* (ca. 1613), fol. 77, in the Royal Library, Copenhagen.

invariably occurred elsewhere in America when Old World epidemic disease was introduced. The virus that caused the death of Huayna Capac was not an isolated one; it was part of a great pandemic that swept vast regions of the Americas. It was likely a continuation of the virus introduced into the Caribbean in 1518 that was carried to the coast of Mesoamerica by the expedition of Pánfilo de Narváez in 1519. Slowly, according to the evidence we have, the infection drifted into the central highlands of Mexico, there too making Spanish conquest of the Aztec empire come with surprising ease. The contagion continued southward into Guatemala, then Nicaragua. At some time it reached Cartagena, Darién, the isthmus of Panama. Foreign sickness leaped ahead of the Spanish, being spread by face-to-face contact between one ethnic entity and another from the north coast of South America upriver.

There is suggestive documentary evidence that disease marched into the highlands of northern South America early. In late September 1530, Nikolaus Federmann reached the Ayamanes in the area of the El Tocuyo River in a spur of the Andes extending into present Venezuela. He relates that elders in the community remembered an illness to which the German adventurer refers as "vioroles" (sic). It had taken its deadly toll years before: "There was a great and general or universal mortality among this nation." So many Indians died as a result that previously inimical groups had joined by marriage, alliance, and confederation. Federmann reports that it seemed that the disease's mortality for them was almost like "our urschlecht [smallpox] although in the Indies there had never been pestilence."[63]

THE ISTHMANIAN CORRIDOR

At some point, smallpox infected the isthmus of Panama and Tierra Firme, then drifted into the interior, being transferred during normal exchange of goods, far ahead of the Europeans. Permanent settlement of the isthmian region began in 1510 with the foundation of Nombre de Dios. Settlements were established on both the Gulf and Pacific coasts, and a small number of permanent residents began to build houses in the towns and to extract whatever of value they could from their nearby Indian allotments. Panama, on the south side of the isthmus, established in 1519, became the starting point for exploration both northward toward Nicaragua and southward along the continen-

---

63 Nikolaus Federmann, *N. Federmanns und H. Stadens Reisen in Südamerica 1529 bis 1555*, ed. Karl Klüpfel (Stuttgart: Literarischer Verein, 1859), pp. 8–9. The word *urschlecht* in fifteenth-century German meant smallpox; see *Matthias Lexers Mittelhochdeutsches Taschenwörterbuch*, 36th ed. (Leipzig: S. Hirzel Verlag, 1980).

tal mainland. Relatively little exploration took place until 1522, when
Pascual de Andagoya sailed southward from Panama. Any illness that
might have been introduced into Panama in the second decade of the
century may have spread by land or on ship toward both north and
south, although our evidence for these early years is only fragmentary.
The European thrust was northward from Panama toward Nicaragua
during the first years of isthmus settlement; from that time, disease
exchange in both directions increased.

Sadly, the isthmus quickly became notorious for its unhealthiness.
Our sources for the epidemic history of the area are incomplete, and
many of the early documents have been lost or destroyed. Nonetheless,
fragmentary information attests to the narrow land body as a focal
point of infection. The heat, heavy rains, marshy coasts, fetid rivers,
and mosquito infestations all led to fevers and elevated mortality.
Oviedo wrote that some 2 million Indians perished in Panama between 1514 and 1530. The historian Antonio de Herrera reported that
more than forty thousand natives lost their lives by disease in Nombre
de Dios and Panama City during a twenty-eight year interval in the
sixteenth century. These numbers are impressionistic and cannot be
the result of actual counts. Nonetheless, they are indicators of a severe
situation. We remember the experience of the settlements at nearby
Darién, beginning in 1514, with horrendous Spanish mortality as-
cribed to *modorra*.

Historians have frequently ignored the extent of pre-Columbian
exchange networks linking Mesoamerica with the Andean world. The
large trade canoe Columbus encountered off the Gulf Coast of Honduras on his fourth voyage suggests the technological capability of the
Taino, Caribs, and their neighbors. Large canoes, with fifteen rows of
paddlers and space for food and goods, permitted exchange between
widely scattered sections of the circum-Caribbean. Even more spectacular was the discovery of large sailing rafts off the Pacific Coast.
Bartolomé Ruiz, pilot during the second attempt of Francisco Pizzaro,
encountered, late in 1526 or early in 1527, large balsa rafts capable of
transport of goods along the Pacific littoral. One raft that carried a sail
and paddle-rudder was from Tumbez, on the northern edge of Inca
Peru. It carried scales to weigh objects, luxury items, precious metals
and stone products, trade ceramics, and fine cotton cloths; these were
probably being exchanged for a number of goods, including the sacred
mullu shells (*Spondylus pictorum*). Although the volume of pre-
Columbian exchange in the region cannot be compared with the trade

in late medieval Europe, it was extensive enough to allow for transfers of both goods and people, as well as pathogens.[64]

Some explorers on Francisco Pizzaro's third expedition became ill in 1531 when they touched on the Ecuadorian coast south of the Bay of Coaque. Friar Pedro Ruiz Navarro wrote that some died "afflicted with smallpox and *bubas.*" Many of those who recovered remained severely disfigured. The term *bubas* could refer to bubonic plague. However, the location of the sores and the impact on the health of the Europeans but not the native Americans leads to the more likely diagnosis of *Verruga peruana.* There was severe bleeding associated with the "reddish boils with the texture of nuts, which form on the face and the nose and in other places." Alternatively, the affliction may have been *pian,* similar in appearance to *verruga* but more akin to syphilis.[65] Nikolaus Federmann mentions that in his campaign in Venezuela a not dissimilar affliction spread among his compatriots as they were marching, at times through swampy districts. The affliction was characterized by fevers and some open sores. Federmann says that they attributed its cause to the water and believed at first that it would not persist, but they became increasingly sick over a period of nine days. Federmann concluded that the true cause was the difficulty of the trip, especially marching on foot through water for four days, a time when they ate weakly seasoned food that was too liquid. In mid-December 1530 they stopped in Hacarygua, where two Christians died. Sickness continued into February 1531 when Federmann decided to march along the coast rather than in the interior. He frequently noted poor food and lack of medicines.[66]

THE SECOND PANDEMIC: MEASLES

The early 1530s marks the first well-documented measles pandemic to sweep the New World. That smallpox and influenza struck first is

---

64 María Rostworowski de Diez Canseco, *Recursos naturales renovables y pesca, siglos XVI y XVII* (Lima: Instituto de Estudios Peruanos, 1981), p. 87; Michael E. Moseley, *The Incas and Their Ancestors* (London: Thames & Hudson, 1992), p. 47.

65 Linda A. Newson, "Old World Epidemics in Early Colonial Ecuador," in *Secret Judgments,* ed. Cook and Lovell, pp. 92–93.

66 Federmann, *Reisen in Südamerica,* pp. 49–50, 68.

Table 2.1. American epidemics, 1518–1533

Dates	Epidemic	Location
1518–28	Smallpox	Caribbean, Mesoamerica, Andes
1530–31	Pneumonic plague, influenza,	
	dolor de costado	Central America
1532–33	Measles	Mesoamerica to Andes

hardly surprising, for influenza does not provide a lifetime immunity, and adults were constantly susceptible to new outbreaks. Smallpox could spread because of the long duration of the infective period of the person suffering the illness and the persistence of the infective agent in the dried scabs given favorable storage conditions. Measles, on the other hand, bestows virtual lifetime immunity on those who contract the malady. That fact, plus the speed of infection and the rapid course of the disease, has to mean that several young people who had never experienced the illness were on board a fleet. The site of original infection could have been Seville, because the population was large enough by the third decade of the sixteenth century for measles to be endemic there. It is possible too, that someone was infected in Seville, and then the illness was transferred to young slaves captured along the African coast. At the same time, given lower population densities in Africa, measles outbreaks there were more sporadic than endemic, with a larger portion of people susceptible during an episode. An infected African slave could have been the source of the first Amerindian disease outbreak. Increasing numbers of young black slaves were forcibly transported to the Caribbean in the 1520s to replace the disappearing native American population. When intro-duced into the vulnerable population of the Americas, measles ex-ploded with exceptional devastation. Survival rates for blacks and Europeans were relatively high, and the disease was frequent and well known to the residents of the Old World. For the native Americans, mortality rates were around 25 to 30 percent, and they continued at these high levels throughout the colonial period.

As was the case with smallpox, measles probably was first intro-duced to the islands of the Caribbean. Dobyns suggests that "perhaps two-thirds of the Indians remaining in Cuba died in an epidemic there in 1529, which may have been the island episode of the measles epidemic."[67] Francisco López de Gómara confused the chronology and source of the measles epidemic as it entered Mexico, referring to events during 1532. "Meanwhile, an epidemic of measles (called by the Indians zahuatltepiton, 'little leprosy') broke out, and many Indians died of it. It was a result of the smallpox brought in by the Negro of Pánfilo de Narváez; it was also a new disease, never seen before in that land."[68] Not only did López de Gómara blame the introduction of smallpox on a single black slave; he compounded the damage by adding measles to the list of imported pathogens introduced by the man.

Toribio de Motolinia argues that measles (sarampión) arrived in Mexico in 1531.[69] Friar Jerónimo de Mendieta said that the epidemic was sarampión, or "small skin rash,"[70] while the report of Domingo Francisco de San Antón Muñón Chimalpahin suggests that it was characterized by a "thin" or "light" rash, and notes that mostly children died. Motolinia even gives the name of the Spaniard who was purported to have transported the disease to the central plateau. Native Americans referred to it as the "small skin rash" to differentiate the disease from the preceding smallpox pandemic. The Chimalpahin report names it zahuatl and describes the symptoms as involving a "thin" or "light" rash, to which children were the primary victims.[71] Overall mortality during the 1531 epidemic according to Motolinia was less than that experienced under the smallpox outbreak of 1519. The following year, 1532, saw either a continuation of the disease or something entirely different. It was referred to in the documents as either zahuatl or totomonaliztli, or a combination. One record indicates that all sectors of the population, including children, were stricken ill. Two sources report that mortality was general, both spatially and in

67 Henry F. Dobyns, "An Outline of Andean Epidemic History to 1720," *Bulletin of the History of Medicine* 37(1963):498; Ramiro Guerra y Sánchez, *Historia de la nación cubana*, 10 vols. (Havana: Editorial Historia de la Nación Cubana, 1952), 1:230.

68 López de Gómara, *Cortés*, p. 397.

69 Toribio de Motolinía o Benavente, *Memoriales o libro de las cosas de la Nueva España y de los naturales dello* (México: UNAM, 1971), p. 22.

70 Fray Jerónimo de Mendieta, *Historia eclesiástica indiana*, 4 vols. (México: Editorial Salvador Chávez Hayhoe, 1945), 4:174.

71 Hanns J. Prem, "Disease Outbreaks in Central Mexico During the Sixteenth Century," in *Secret Judgments*, ed. Cook and Lovell, pp. 27–28; Domingo Francisco de San Antón Muñón Chimalpahin, "Die Relationen Chimalpahins zur Geschichte Mexicos," *Das Jahrhundert nach der Conquista* (Hamburg: Cram de Gruyter, 1965), pp. 7–8.

terms of the people infected. In some locales many older people died, which suggests it was not a recurrence of smallpox, unless that region had been spared a decade before. Given the confusion in the native sources, it is probable that we see the appearance of one, or more likely two, new non-American diseases in central Mexico in 1531–32.[72]

The expedition of 1530–31 under Diego de Guzmán is associated with the introduction of one or more foreign pathogens into Nueva Galicia. According to Reff, an epidemic (malaria, typhoid, or dysentery) decimated Guzmán's native allies and the province of Aztatlan around September 1530. Measles extended along the western coast of Mexico in 1534 from Nayarit into Sinaloa. Reports suggest that 130,000 natives succumbed from measles and "bloody stools." Reff identifies dysentery or typhoid as possible causes associated with the high number of deaths.[73]

Lovell documented more important evidence for Guatemala, citing a letter of Pedro de Alvarado dated 1 September 1532, to the king, sent from Santiago de Guatemala: "Throughout New Spain, there passed a sickness which they say is measles, which struck the Indians and swept the land, leaving it totally empty. It arrived in this province some three months ago [i.e., June of 1532]." The bout clearly continued to spread, for Royal Treasurer Pedro de los Ríos wrote to the ruler on 22 June 1533, complaining that there were not enough Indian workers for the placer mines because of the "many sicknesses which have struck them, especially one recently of measles." Alvarado, a conquistador not known for acts of charity, claimed that he had taken action to assist the natives, "to better cure them, and not allow them to die in such numbers as everywhere else." But his efforts were largely in vain, for "many are dead."[74] The governor continued, saying that he had removed ill slaves from the mines in order to assist in their cure and that he had also ordered encomenderos to provide medications and food for their charges until they were well, without extracting the normal labor services. It is precisely at this time that ships and men were being prepared to join in the conquest of Peru.[75]

72 Prem, "Disease Outbreaks," pp. 27–31.
73 Daniel T. Reff, "Contact Shock in Northwestern New Spain, 1518–1764," in *Disease and Demography in the Americas*, ed. John W. Verano and Douglas H. Ubelaker (Washington, DC: Smithsonian Institution Press, 1992), p. 266.
74 Lovell, "Disease and Depopulation," p. 70.
75 Raúl Porras Barrenechea, *Cartas del Perú (1524–1543)* (Lima: Sociedad de Bibliófilos Peruanos, 1959), pp. 31–33; and Lovell, "Disease and Depopulation," pp. 69–70.

The diagnosis of disease in Central America in the early 1530s is complicated by descriptions of symptoms that indicate measles as well as other illnesses, including smallpox and the plague. Hernán Méndez de Sotomayor, a witness in the later administrative review of Pedro de Alvarado, commented that "in this province, both on the coast and inland, there has been much illness amongst the natives from disease and respiratory infection [romadizos] and measles, and this has played a part in the loss of so many Indian lives."[76] Newson reports bubonic plague in early 1531 in Nicaragua, followed by measles in 1533.[77] Lovell notes "sickness" in Guatemala in 1533, and MacLeod reports generalized measles in Central America from 1532 to 1534.[78] Newson concurs in her records of the disease experience of Honduras and Nicaragua.[79] Actually, the documentary report of passage of the first great smallpox pandemic through Honduras and Nicaragua comes several years after the event, in 1527. In administrative orders of 7 October 1527 to agents in the city of Granada, it was reported that the Indians had already been decimated by a previous epidemic of smallpox. Panama City, Nata, and the Port of Honduras were authorized to import slaves to compensate for the labor shortage. Two years later, another document notes that the mines of Gracias a Dios and San Andrés were running out of workers because of "figo [higo] y enfermedades." Many Indians died, along with some Europeans.[80] Covarrubias defines higo as "the illness that is commonly called morana [almorrana] because of its similarity with the fig." In modern Spanish almorrana refers to "bloody hemorrhoids." In the early seventeenth century Covarrubias noted four forms: with blood, without blood, with crack or split, and almorrana of sodomites. Murdo MacLeod says it may have been pneumonic plague.[81] There is evidence that bubonic and pneumonic plague erupted in Nicaragua in 1531. Castañeda wrote on

76 Wendy Kramer, *Encomienda Politics in Early Colonial Guatemala, 1524–1544* (Boulder, CO: Westview Press, 1994), p. 114; original from Archivo General de Indias, Seville, Justicia 295.

77 Linda A. Newson, "The Depopulation of Nicaragua in the Sixteenth Century," *Journal of Latin American Studies* 14(1982):279–80.

78 Murdo J. MacLeod, *Spanish Central America: A Socioeconomic History, 1520–1720* (Berkeley: University of California Press, 1973), p. 98.

79 Linda A. Newson, *The Cost of Conquest: Indian Decline in Honduras under Spanish Rule* (Boulder, CO: Westview Press, 1986), pp. 128–29; idem, *Indian Survival in Colonial Nicaragua* (Norman: University of Oklahoma Press, 1987), p. 120.

80 Newson, *Indian Survival in Nicaragua*, p. 119.

81 MacLeod, *Spanish Central America*, p. 98.

30 May 1531 that two-thirds of the Indians had buboes and that most of the infected Indians lived in Spanish houses. In the León district, Indians were dying from "stomach pains and fevers," and "pains in the stomach and sides" that he referred to as *landres*. The term *landres* as it was used in Spain at the time was a fairly sure bet to have been the plague, with most individuals contracting the bubonic form, but with occasional bloody and deadly cases of pneumonic plague in some households or in villages.[82] It is tragic that a measles epidemic, beginning in 1532, was rampant so soon afterward.

Antonio de Herrera wrote that "at this time there was such a great epidemic of measles in the Province of Honduras spreading from house to house and village to village, that many people died; and although the disease also affected the Spaniards, . . . none of them died. . . . This same disease of measles and dysentery (*camaras de sangre*) passed to Nicaragua where also many Indians died . . . and two years ago there was a general epidemic of pleurisy [*dolor de costado*] and stomach pains which also carried away many Indians."[83] On 28 April Pedro de los Ríos wrote the emperor from the city of León that he had recently arrived to assume office as treasury agent. He had discovered many of the settlers in debt and gold production stalled because many "had died from illness, especially measles; lately so many Indians have died that some *vecinos* have none. Others have removed their Indians from the mines because they continue to die."[84] Oviedo provides very similar information for Honduras, arguing that measles and other illnesses had caused the death of about one-half the inhabitants; "the most susceptible were those who were servants in Spanish households or workers on Spanish estates."[85]

Conditions in Central America during the immediate years following the conquest of New Spain were especially trying for the native Americans. Several groups of marauding conquistadores marched back and forth across the area, searching for elusive treasure. Most found little of immediate worth, and the Europeans took the only thing of value – human slaves to be used elsewhere, on the estates of the islands of the Caribbean, or as auxiliaries in the conquest of Peru.

82 Newson, *Indian Survival in Nicaragua*, pp. 119–20.
83 Ibid., p. 120; Newson, *Cost of Conquest*, p. 129; Antonio de Herrera y Tordesillas, *Historia general de los hechos de los castellanos en las islas y tierra firme del mar océano*, 17 vols. (Madrid: Real Academia de la Historia, 1934), 10:72.
84 Porras Barrenechea, *Cartas*, pp. 46–47.
85 Newson, *Cost of Conquest*, p. 129.

The very close contacts between Nicaragua and Panama, as men prepared for the Peruvian expeditions in the early 1530s, meant that any epidemic could be quickly transferred to the south. We have noted variations in identification of the illness that killed Huayna Capac. It is possible that the confusion is a consequence of a second epidemic that swept the region prior to Atahualpa's capture by Francisco Pizarro at the highland center of Cajamarca. There was an epidemic on the isthmus of Panama that could have easily been transferred southward, given the nature of the hectic preparations for the conquest of Peru. In a letter to Charles V, Licentiate de la Gama wrote from Nombre de Dios on the Caribbean side of the isthmus on 24 May 1531, reporting that the entire region was afflicted by disease. "From a ship that has arrived from Nicaragua the pestilence has struck this land, and it has been so great that although it has not yet ended, two parts of all the people that there are in this land have died, native Indians as well as slaves, and among them some Christians. I attest to Your Majesty that it is the most frightening thing that I have ever seen, because even the strongest does not last more than a day and a half, and some two or three hours, and now it reigns as at the beginning, and has become concentrated in Panama. The clerics are organizing processions, and praying, but not even these pleas to Our Lord have lifted his ire, to the point that I do not think there will remain alive a single person in all the land."[86]

De la Gama also complained that there was not a doctor or a pharmacy in the area. In early September, the town council of the city of Panama notified the ruler that few Indians remained after the passage of the pestilence, and they requested permission to use Indians from Nicaragua, Tumbez, and Peru, unwittingly condemning them to death.[87] In September of the following year, measles was noted as having arrived in Santiago de Guatemala from New Spain, but there is no indication that this was the outbreak experienced in Panama in 1531. Indeed, the speed of death, and the fact that all segments of the population were liable to become infected in the Panamanian isthmus epidemic of 1531, indicates it was not measles.[88] The mention of *landres* in the account of Central America is the best evidence we have that this may have been an outbreak of the pneumonic plague. In September 1531, the cabildo of the city of Panama notified the king that few Indians remained after the passage of the pestilence, and

---

86 Porras Barrenechea, *Cartas*, p. 22.   87 Ibid., p. 24.   88 Ibid., p. 33.

he requested permission to use Indian slaves from Nicaragua, Tumbez, and Peru proper.[89] Belalcázar provided numerous reinforcements from Nicaragua in 1532, and in 1533 Francisco de Godoy continued to send Nicaraguan contingents. Large numbers of Nicaraguan slaves were taken and used for the Andean venture.[90] Much later, Lizárraga reported that the Indians near Lima had failed to block the Spanish, partly because several years before there had swept through the region an epidemic of *romadizo* and *dolor de costado* "which carried off the greater part of them."[91]

Accurate diagnosis of the early 1530s series of illnesses that so devastated native American peoples is complicated partly by the fact that in 1531 a number of Spanish explorers of the northwestern coast of South America became ill and severely disfigured, and, as we have already noted, some of them died. Newson suggests that this sickness was *Verruga peruana*. Licentiate Tomás Lópes, in his "Tratado de los tres elementos," described in detail the symptoms displayed by the Europeans. He reported that even as the first Spanish reached Puerto Viejo, they fell ill with "a sickness of a certain kind of smallpox or blisters [*ampollas*], that afflicts them in the whole face, especially in the eyes, and of it some die, and others are left blind and there are few or none at all who escape without feeling this infirmity, and it occurred so quickly that merely upon entering that place it struck them."[92]

The second epidemic wave of the early 1530s to sweep the isthmus may have included measles and one or more disease elements such as pneumonic plague and influenza; the complex nature of the epidemic experience helps to explain the confusion in the later accounts of the death of Huayna Capac. By the 1560s and 1570s, most of those who remembered the Andean land before the arrival of the Europeans were unable to distinguish the 1524–25 epidemic from that of 1531 or 1533. All three epidemic cycles may have taken place before the appearance of the foreigners. The arrival of the outsiders and the capture of

89 Ibid., p. 24.
90 James Lockhart, *Spanish Peru, 1532–1560: A Colonial Society* (Madison: University of Wisconsin Press, 1968); David R. Radell, "The Indian Slave Trade and Population of Nicaragua during the Sixteenth Century," in *The Native Population of the Americas in 1492*, 2d ed., ed. William M. Denevan (Madison: University of Wisconsin Press, 1992), pp. 67–76.
91 Reginaldo de Lizárraga, *Descripción de las Indias* (Lima: Pequeños Grandes Libros de Historia Americana, 1946), p. 40.
92 Manuscript Collection of the Real Academia de la Historia, Madrid, document A/69 4806, 134v.

Atahualpa at Cajamarca were watersheds in the chronological cosmos of Andean peoples. In Andean cosmology these events mark what is called the Pachacutec, the great upheaval, the overturning of the world. The most astute native witnesses would have had to be born before 1510, and by 1570 they would have been more than sixty years old. Many, if not most, of the trained quipucamayos died during the first pandemics, and most imperial records became unintelligible with the demise of the record keepers. Disappearance of the quipus resulted in the loss of an accurate account of the Andean past.

If epidemic wave followed epidemic wave, sweeping inland from the Caribbean shore, then the cumulative demographic impact on the peoples of the continent must have been massive. Dobyns suggests, for example, that measles extended as far as Florida, perhaps even beyond, in 1531–33.[93] The spread of epidemics was not constrained by artificial political boundaries; even natural frontiers often provided no obstacle to the passage of epidemic infection. Sixteenth-century efforts at establishing quarantine to prevent the appearance of the plague almost inevitably ended in dismal failure. Disease, once introduced, tended to run its course unabated until the pool of susceptible victims was reduced to the point at which the epidemic naturally died out. Both in the case of the initial smallpox pandemic and the subsequent measles occurrence, Old World viral infections were acting on a population that had never experienced either disease before. Epidemics among virgin populations evolve in ways different from what is expected when they act on peoples that have been exposed to them for generations. High virulence is often the result.[94] Such seems to have been the case with the initial smallpox and measles epidemics that swept the New World. Dobyns argues that the first great smallpox pandemic was not confined to Mesoamerica and the Andean region but that it must have spread far afield into Florida and the interior of North America. Written evidence, the true foundation for establishing historical veracity, is incomplete. Archaeological evidence that might verify or disprove the massive impact of the initial epidemics of smallpox and measles is spotty and difficult to evaluate. Recent work by Ramenofsky points to the possibility of a massive die-off of native

93 Henry F. Dobyns, *Their Number Become Thinned: Native American Population Dynamics in Eastern North America* (Knoxville: University of Tennessee Press, 1983), pp. 270, 284–85.

94 Thomas M. Whitmore, *Disease and Death in Early Colonial Mexico: Simulating Amerindian Depopulation* (Boulder, CO: Westview Press, 1992), pp. 52–59.

Americans in part of what is now the United States "around 1500," or at the time of initial contact.[95] Clearly, further investigation needs to be undertaken before we can completely evaluate the nature and impact of the dissemination of the first great pandemics of the sixteenth century on the vulnerable native American population.

95 Ann F. Ramenofsky, *Vectors of Death: The Archaeology of European Contact* (Albuquerque: University of New Mexico Press, 1987).

CHAPTER THREE

SETTLING IN

EPIDEMICS AND CONQUEST
TO THE END OF THE FIRST CENTURY

This contagious malady ran everywhere so strangely that several
of us died of it, and an infinite number of savages.

André Thevet, Villegagnon's colony, Rio de Janeiro, 1556

From Mexico has entered . . . a plague of smallpox and typhus,
from which have died, and die daily still, a great number of
Indians, especially young children.

Pedro de Villalobos, Audiencia of Guatemala, 1577

The wilde people at first comminge of our men died verie fast
and said amongest themselues, It was the Englisshe God that
made them die so faste.

Primrose log, Drake's fleet, St. Augustine, 1586

By 1542, a half century after the arrival of the denizens of the Old
World in the Americas, Hispaniola was devastated, and severe depopulation had commenced on surrounding islands in the Caribbean and
on the nearby mainland. The foreign pathogens were active, winnowing the people more quickly even than the sword or arquebus
could, and certainly much more silently and effectively. The first
sicknesses of 1493 had been followed by others even more deadly. In
the second decade of the sixteenth century, smallpox directly aided
the Spanish conquest of the Aztec empire and may have killed the
Inca ruler long before Europeans set foot in the land of Tawantinsuyu.
In both Mesoamerica and the Andes, the death of a ruler and large
numbers of subjects from sickness contributed to a fatal weakness,
perhaps even a loss of the will to resist the invaders. By 1533 influenza,
smallpox, and measles, three of the deadliest airborne communicable

diseases, had swept the New World. Malaria too was introduced, and in subsequent decades other diseases sequentially made their appearance. By the end of the first century after contact, most Old World diseases had taken their excruciating toll of Amerindians.

Smallpox and measles were two of the most deadly epidemic diseases. Both had afflicted Europeans and Africans for generations; they were endemic in southern Europe and North Africa and were predominantly childhood diseases. The ports of Andalusia, from which most of the early voyages initiated, were hit by epidemic after epidemic. Seville in 1500 was already a large city by early modern European standards, and by 1580 its population had surged to over 100,000, large enough for many communicable diseases to remain endemic.[1] Most sailors were old enough to have been exposed to smallpox and measles before they first sailed. Hence, it must have been several years before a person boarded ship who had never experienced the disease before. Yet someone became infected by the virus, fell ill, and then transmitted it to another susceptible person, in a chain, until the deadly cargo was unloaded on the shores of the opposite side of the Atlantic. Initial mortality was high for "virgin" populations; Duffy notes that as late as the eighteenth century smallpox epidemics carried away 55 to 80 percent of Amerindians infected in eastern North America.[2] The introduction of measles was also delayed but was deadly when it came at last. The spread and impact of influenza is distinct. In various forms it mutated with facility; one influenza episode afforded the individual little protection for a later epidemic occurrence. Other diseases were transmitted by intermediate vectors; typhus, bubonic plague, yellow fever, and malaria were the most significant of these. With the arthropod-transmitted infections, a whole series of complex factors were brought into play before an epidemic stage was reached and the disease took lasting root in the Americas. The etiology of plague and typhus made for large variations in speed of spread and localized mortality. Plague exists in climates with temperatures within the range of 10° to 30° C, with the bubonic form being more pervasive at the higher temperatures and the pneumonic variety in the cooler regions. Typhus is most potent where it is generally cool, where woolen and linen clothing is layered and tends to become quickly dirty, places

---

1 Noble David Cook and José Hernández Palomo, "Epidemias en Triana (Sevilla, 1660–1865)," *Annali della facolta di Economia e Commercio della Universita di Bari* 31(1992):53–81.

2 John Duffy, *Epidemics in Colonial America* (Baton Rouge: Louisiana State University Press, 1953), p. 244.

where body lice are most prevalent. In tropical regions where bathing occurs daily and clothing is minimal among the Amerindian population, typhus appears less frequently.[3] Thus, it is not surprising that the airborne epidemics – measles, smallpox, and influenza – were probably the first deadly killers in the New World, doing their damage for at least a generation before typhus and the plague became fully acclimated to the new environment around the middle of the sixteenth century.

TERRIBLE DEATHS OF THE MID-1540s

Two, perhaps three major epidemic series swept large sections of the Americas between the mid-1540s and the end of the century. Several observers report that a terrible sickness broke out in central Mexico in 1545. Prem argues that it was "probably the most disastrous" of all epidemics to assault the area during the course of the sixteenth century.[4] Yet surprisingly, in spite of its severity, there are only a few descriptions of the symptoms. Perhaps the lacunae can be accounted for by the fact that it killed quickly or that the symptoms never progressed to distinguishable rashes. The infection was widespread, and it persisted until 1548. The sickness may have been introduced by the fleet of Bartolomé de Las Casas. One of the best descriptions of this epidemic period in Mesoamerica comes from the Dominican, Friar Tomás de la Torre, who kept a detailed diary of his voyage from Salamanca, Spain, to Ciudad Real de Chiapa in New Spain in 1544–45.

Twenty-six ships set out, crossing the sandbar at Sanlúcar de Barrameda on 10 July 1544. The fleet included Bartolomé de Las Casas, who was returning to the Indies to assume his post as bishop of Chiapas. As was customary in many prior expeditions to the Indies, the fleet spent ten days (20–29 July) on the island of Gomera, taking on supplies and repairing the ships. The fleet sailed into the Caribbean on 27 August 1544. Friar de la Torre must have been well instructed on the plight of Amerindian peoples by their protector Bartolomé de

3 Linda A. Newson, *The Cost of Conquest: Indian Decline in Honduras under Spanish Rule* (Boulder, CO: Westview Press, 1986), p. 313; Percy M. Ashburn, *The Ranks of Death: A Medical History of the Conquest of America* (New York: Coward-McCann, 1947), pp. 81, 95–96; and Hans Zinsser, *Rats, Lice and History* (New York: Bantam Books, 1960), pp. 261–62.

4 Hanns J. Prem, "Disease Outbreaks in Central Mexico during the Sixteenth Century," in *The Secret Judgments of God: Native Peoples and Old World Disease in Colonial Spanish America*, ed. Noble David Cook and W. George Lovell (Norman: University of Oklahoma Press, 1992), p. 31.

Las Casas, for Torre wrote in his diary that "before these islands were the most populous in the world; but the majority of them were assaulted by the insatiable greed and the extraordinary cruelty and tyranny of the Spaniards." In Puerto Rico the fleet split up. It was there that Torre first noted shipboard mortality in his diary: "Many people had already died."[5]

Finally, on 9 September the friar and his group disembarked at Santo Domingo. There were fifty-two in the company, not counting Las Casas and his men, and considerable strain was put on the resources of the monasteries at Santo Domingo to feed them. Furthermore, "some also became ill there . . . the royal officials did all they could to assist the sick . . . the healthy served the ill with great charity." Although some of the men were very ill, no one died, or if someone did, the death was not mentioned by Torre. The group remained in Santo Domingo until mid-December, then continued to the Mesoamerican coast at Campeche.[6]

Campeche was at the time a port with about 500 houses, according to the diarist. From there a smaller group continued to Tabasco on a much overloaded small coastal vessel, which was hit by a strong storm from the north. They were shipwrecked, and several of the friar's companions drowned. Some survivors walked back along the coast to Campeche, but twenty remained on the Isle de los Términos awaiting rescue. Increasingly, de la Torre complained about mosquitoes; one night they returned to sleep on the ship because of the "infinite number of mosquitoes on the shore." On the island Torre says, "In order to free ourselves of the mosquitoes we burned much of the undergrowth, and also the tents that they gave us, among other things, in Campeche." At another point he lamented the bothersome insects: "We thought that they were going to eat us alive." Only when the sea wind was strong enough did they disappear. Friar Cristóbal went about "with a sheepskin over his head, with two holes for eyes cut out, because of the mosquitoes." There Friar Pedro Calvo fell ill, "from some pains in the bowels that doubled him up and tied him into knots, from which we thought he could never be cured or ever retrieve his fortunes, but after many months he was cured of all."[7]

The hungry mosquitoes swarmed in such numbers that at night the men could get relief only by covering their bare feet and arms with a

5 Tomás de la Torre, *Diario de viaje de Salamanca a Chiapa, 1544–1545* (Caleruega [Burgos]: Editorial OPE, 1985), pp. 74, 76.
6 Ibid., p. 9.   7 Ibid., pp. 122, 125, 126.

mud pack, and even then the mosquitoes bit them with such ferocity that they were forced to flee and throw themselves into the sea to escape. On 6 February 1545 they reached Xicalango, and Friar de la Torre reported "there were many long-beaked mosquitoes, and we took great advantage of the sleeping nets that we brought, for without them sleep would have been virtually impossible. . . . The legs of the vicar and Friar Diego Hernández were so swollen by the bites of the mosquitoes that it was a pitiful thing to see, because this type of mosquito is very poisonous and causes swelling when there are many bites." One group reached Tabasco by 13 February, but within two days "the friars began to find themselves ill, because the village is very unhealthy." From there they walked primarily overland toward Chiapas, facing constant hunger and insect pests. By late February Friar Tomás de San Juan had fallen ill, and "the father vicar was also feverish and indisposed." The group stayed briefly in the house of Pedro Gentil and his wife, who had settled there. De la Torre and the others were delighted as they entered the house and saw "the tables set with German damask tablecloths reaching to the floor, and on top many glasses and porcelains with abundant bread and melons of Castile." They joyously thanked their hosts "for the abundant meal and drink, not of cacao, but of a most excellent wine from Guadalcanal." Shortly thereafter Friar Rodrigo fell ill, although he was not in mortal danger.[8]

Here diarist de la Torre ended his complaints about insect infestations. Perhaps the mosquitoes became less bothersome as the brothers continued inland. At the same time, sickness increasingly consumed his attention. On 3 March they had to assist Friar Tomás de San Juan as well as "the father vicar, who although still on foot, by then had a fever and was constantly falling and getting up." Next, Friars Jerónimo de San Vicente, Jorge de León, and Alonso de Norena became sick. Particularly difficult was the ascent of Tlapilula; some were so ill they crawled upward on all fours. On 6 March they rested. Friars Juan Cabrera and Luis de Cuenca arrived with supplies that had been left at Pedro Gentil's house. A servant named Segovia and his cousin Roldán, "a youth and most vigorous," had been left behind and eventually died. A servant named Nuñez had been left to guard some provisions in Tlapilula, where he too became ill. The friars took him into Pedro Gentil's house "where he took leave of his senses emitting, through the nose, an infinite number of maggots [gusanos]." Friar Tomás seems to have become ill himself: "The same day that we rested

8 Ibid., pp. 130–33, 136, 151, 152.

many of us fell ill; I do not know how many there were of us, except that there was no one left to serve anyone. I think that there were thirteen of us strewn about the hut; three on the mattress of the cleric, and the rest on the ground; all with fever in a forsaken place." The next day (7 March) they resumed their trek, even though many were feverish. De la Torre said that the stomach pains of Pedro Calvo were then so intense that he could not raise his head from his knees. "It was pitiful to see him, and we thought he would die." Friar Alonso Portillo had to be carried in a litter on the friars' shoulders, and at times they "had to carry Friar Alonso on their backs." As the journey progressed, the men were tested continually by lack of food, excessive heat, thirst, and persistent illness. Bartolomé de las Casas had already reached Chiapas. Apprised of the plight of the group, he had sent by horse some supplies, which much comforted the friars. Finally in mid-March 1545, after a three-month ordeal, the group was met by Bishop Las Casas as it entered the Ciudad Real de Chiapa. According to the diarist, many continued to experience fevers as they settled in.[9]

The arrival of the friars coincided with the appearance in Mexico of one of the most deadly disease outbreaks in the sixteenth century. The native peoples of central Mexico called the disease *cocoliztli*, or *hueycocoliztli*, meaning "sickness," or "great sickness."[10] Some native sources indicate that symptoms included fever and bleeding from the eyes, mouth, nose, and anus. The Spanish observer Mendieta mentions its "full bloodiness," referring to the heavy bloody nasal discharge.[11] Debate continues over the accurate identification of the epidemic, although there seems to be a consensus that falls on *Typhus exanthematicus*. Alexander von Humboldt identified the sickness as "typhus-like," and Sticker called it *Typhus exanthematicus*.[12] Zinnser concluded that it was typhus, whereas McNeill and Dobyns are somewhat reserved.[13] Prem, after careful evaluation of the sources, con-

9 Ibid., pp. 154, 155, 160–61.
10 Elsa Malvido and Carlos Viesca, "La epidemia de cocoliztli de 1576," *Historias* (Mexico) 11(1985):27.
11 Prem, "Disease Outbreaks in Central Mexico," p. 32.
12 Alexander Freiherr von Humboldt, *Ensayo político sobre el reino de la Nueva España* (México: Editorial Porrúa, 1966), pp. 45, 513; George Sticker, "Die Einschleppung europaischer Krankheiten in Amerika während der Entdeckungszeit; ihr Einfluss auf den Rückgang der Bevölkerung," *Ibero-Amerikanisches Archiv* 6(1932):205; and Prem, "Disease Outbreaks in Central Mexico," p. 32.
13 Zinnser, *Rats, Lice, and History*, p. 256; William H. McNeill, *Plagues and Peoples* (Garden City, NY: Anchor Doubleday, 1976), p. 185; and Henry F.

cludes that "even though typhus remains the most satisfactory explanation, doubts persist."[14] It also might have been pulmonary plague, as
MacLeod postulates for Guatemala.[15]

Shortly after the deadly epidemic of the mid-1540s swept central
Mesoamerica, an important medical text (1552) was compiled by an
Indian doctor, Martín de la Cruz. It was translated into Latin by a
native from Xochimilco named Juan Badiano under the title *Libellus
de medicinalibus indorum herbis*. This brilliantly illustrated work describes the therapeutic value of certain animals, plants, and minerals.[16]
Cures are provided for a variety of complaints, including hemorrhoids,
burns, scabies, epilepsy, heavy menstruation, skull fractures, headaches,
angina, sore throat, and many others. The cure of fever illustrates the
potential importance of the book as a text of native medical lore and
probably reflects the symptoms of the mid-1540s series of illnesses:
"The face of the feverish person takes on many aspects. At times it
becomes red, sometimes black, and other times it becomes pallid.
Blood is spit up. There is vomit. The body becomes agitated and
moves to and fro. One sees little. The mouth senses at times, especially
in the palate, bitterness, burning, and sometimes sweetness. The stomach generally is very upset. If the danger is not dealt with when the
urine is white, clear, or milkish, it will be too late to prepare the
medications." Martín de la Cruz suggested that great assistance could
be provided if one ground a number of native herbs together: *centson-
xochitl, teoiztaquilitl, aquiztli, tlanextia, xihuitl, cuauhtlahuitzquilitl, tonat-
iuh ixiuh*.[17]

Juan Bautista de Pomar, writing about the people of Tetzcoco in
central Mexico in 1582, reported the passage of several *pestilencias
generales* in earlier years. At the time he wrote his description, one
epidemic that began in 1575 and was rampant for seven years continued to take its victims, just as one had approximately forty years earlier
(ca. 1542). Both Indian and Spanish doctors diligently attempted to
find a cure but could not. They called the illness *cocoliztli ezahualhu-*

Dobyns, "An Outline of Andean Epidemic History to 1720," *Bulletin of the
History of Medicine* 37 (1963):499.

14 Prem, "Disease Outbreaks in Central Mexico," p. 34.
15 Murdo MacLeod, *Spanish Central America: A Socioeconomic History, 1520–
1720* (Berkeley: University of California Press, 1973), p. 19.
16 Alfredo López Austin, *Textos de medicina nahuatl* (México: UNAM, 1975), p.
40, examines the contribution of Martín de la Cruz.
17 Ibid., pp. 96–97.

acque, meaning a pestilence of gloomy and brown-colored fury (*pesti-lencia de colera adusta y requemada*). Juan Bautista de Pomar said that indeed it was an appropriate label, "because most who died expelled from their mouth a humor like putrified blood."

Bautista de Pomar also suggested that remedies could alleviate suffering and mortality that came with certain diseases, at least those to which the native American death rate was similar to that of the outsiders. These sicknesses included mumps (*paperas*) and hemorrhages (*flujos de sangre*).[18] According to Bautista de Pomar, none of these was as contagious or as deadly as the great epidemics. "And they also tend to have *tabardete* [typhus] and *dolor de costado* [*pleurisy*] and *camaras de sangre* [dysentery]. And as all these illnesses are known by the Span-iards, they have cured and treated according to their rule and opinion, applying the medicines and ordinary treatments which are still used at the present time." Juan Bautista de Pomar found that nothing was effective against the ravages of the worst killers. "For the *cocoliztles,* no remedy has been found." The only people who might find recompense were "the rich people, dressed, well covered, and well fed, and those who lived in the warmer lands [*tierras cálidas*]." He concluded that those suffering most were the poor who lived in cool, dry regions, and he lamented that "no one could find out the secret and mystery of why this was so."[19]

All sources concur that the death rate from the sickness was horren-dous. It afflicted all segments of the population, although native Americans seem hardest hit. Motolinia reported a death rate of 60 to 90 percent. In Tlaxcala, up to 1,000 fell daily, and the total number of deaths reached 150,000. At Cholula, 1,000 may have died.[20] Friar Bernardino de Sahagún claims to have interred 10,000 in the modest town of Tlatelolco. He himself fell ill near the end of the epidemic.[21] Torquemada, referring to a wide geographical area, estimated that 800,000 died from the disease.[22] McCaa argues that the death rate for the 1545 epidemic was probably the highest of the century, although

18 Ibid., pp. 138–39.   19 Ibid.
20 Toribio de Motolinía o Benavente, *Memoriales o libro de las cosas de la Nueva España y de los naturales dello* (México: UNAM, 1971), p. 413.
21 Bernardino de Sahagún, *Florentine Codex: General History of the Things of New Spain,* ed. Arthur J. O. Anderson and Charles E. Dibble, 13 in 12 vols. (Santa Fe, NM: School of American Research, 1954), 3:356.
22 Juan de Torquemada, *Monarquía indiana* (Madrid: Rodríguez Franco, 1723), 1:642; Prem, "Disease Outbreaks in Central Mexico," pp. 33–34.

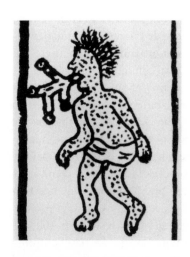

Figure 3.1. Depiction of Mexican ill in 1545 with *cocoliztli* (*Typhus exanthematicus*, or pneumonic plague), from *Codex en Cruz*.

because the population was greater in 1519, the actual number who died from the first smallpox pandemic could have been larger than the number who succumbed from typhus.[23] From 1545 to 1548, western Mexico from Nayarit through central Sinaloa was hit by sicknesses, probably typhus. The discovery of major mineral deposits in Zacatecas in 1546 led to continuous infection in and around the center, according to Reff.[24]

The 1545–48 sicknesses also afflicted Guatemala. At the time, the Audiencia capital was at Gracias a Dios, in what is today western Honduras. The members of the Audiencia had notice of the devastation being caused by the epidemic in Mexico, but as late as 1 December 1545 wrote the monarch that the pestilence still "has not reached Guatemala."[25] When it did arrive, it was called *gucumatz*, and it was deadly. Most contemporaries reported that the pestilence had come from Mexico and had extracted a heavy human toll as it moved forward. The settler and encomendero Gonzalo de Ortiz wrote to the Crown that "God sent down such sickness upon the Indians that three out of every four of them perished," and that "because of this, all is

23 Robert McCaa, "Spanish and Nahuatl Views on Smallpox and Demographic Catastrophe in Mexico," *Journal of Interdisciplinary History* 25(1995):427–28.
24 Daniel T. Reff, *Disease, Depopulation, and Culture Change in Northwestern New Spain, 1518–1764* (Salt Lake City: University of Utah Press, 1991), pp. 266–67.
25 W. George Lovell, "Disease and Depopulation in Early Colonial Guatemala," in *Secret Judgments*, ed. Cook and Lovell, p. 72.

now lost in Mexico, and here also."[26] The late seventeenth-century Guatemalan chronicler Francisco Antonio de Fuentes y Guzmán, writing in the *Recordación Florida*, reports that around this time there was "typhus, or chills and fevers [malaria?], a common epidemic of the coast."[27] As with Mexico, accurate diganosis of the Guatemalan episode is difficult. Both MacLeod and Orellana equate the Quiche term *k'ucumatz* with pneumonic plague.[28] The symptoms of pneumonic plague and *Typhus exanthematicus*, which both overwhelm the human respiratory system, are virtually indistinguishable. Unable to identify the 1545 outbreak conclusively, Newson concludes that it could have been either pneumonic plague or typhus. She found no evidence that it spread farther south.[29]

The original source of the 1540s epidemic must have been the Old World. Indeed, typhus was widely distributed in the Iberian peninsula in the mid-1540s. According to Hampe Martínez, an epidemic ravaged central Spain in 1545. As a consequence of various deaths in Valladolid, the Court was shifted southward to Madrid. Cardinal Tavera succumbed to epidemic disease on 5 August 1545. The following year in northern Castile, in the region between Burgos and León, some people were reported ill with *dolor de costado*. *Dolor de costado* has been variously translated as "chest pain," or "pain in the side," but perhaps the most appropriate definition is "pain in the rib cage." The term reflects upper respiratory discomfort, as with severe infections involving the lungs and chest cavity, when pain that is difficult to locate exactly pierces one when the thorax expands and contracts as the lungs inhale and exhale. The pain might be reported in the back, the chest, the side, the ribs. The English used the word *pleurisy* to describe the same affliction. Both Iberian and Anglo physicians relied on Greek medical knowledge. *Pleury* is the plural for rib; it "also refers to the

26 Archivo General de Indias, Seville, Justicia 299; Lovell, "Disease in Early Colonial Guatemala," p. 71.
27 Lovell, "Disease in Early Colonial Guatemala," p. 72; W. George Lovell, *Conquest and Survival in Colonial Guatemala: A Historical Geography of the Cuchumatán Highlands, 1500–1821*, rev. ed. (Montreal and Kingston: McGill-Queens University Press, 1992), p. 183.
28 Lovell, "Disease in Early Colonial Guatemala," p. 72; MacLeod, *Spanish Central America*, p. 19; and Sandra L. Orellana, *Indian Medicine in Highland Guatemala* (Albuquerque: University of New Mexico Press, 1987), pp. 143, 146.
29 Linda A. Newson, "The Depopulation of Nicaragua in the Sixteenth Century," *Journal of Latin American Studies* 14(1982):120.

side or body wall containing the ribs. The Greek term *pleuodynia* means pain in the chest's wall, and *pleuritis* means disease there.[30] Diagnosis is imprecise: Those afflicted may have had influenza, typhus, pneumonia, or even a form of the plague. The unity lies in the symptoms: pains in the rib cage.

Licentiate Pedro de la Gasca, sent by Charles V with a fleet of ten ships to quell the uprising of the Peruvian encomenderos under Gonzalo Pizarro, himself fell ill of fevers on the island of Gomera in mid-1546. The expeditionary force had left Sanlúcar on 26 May 1546 and provisioned on Gomera in the Canaries. The passage across the Atlantic was relatively good, and they landed in Santa Marta on the Colombian coast on 10 July. There the licentiate learned of the death of the first Peruvian viceroy, Blasco Núñez Vela, in a battle against the rebels, giving Gasca's mission of pacification an even greater urgency. He left Santa Marta on 15 July with his fleet, and on 27 July reached Nombre de Dios, and finally Panama on 13 August.[31]

Health conditions on the isthmus of Panama were terrible for both natives and Europeans. Oviedo knew the region well and described its horrors. Pedro de Cieza de León, who passed through for the first time in the early 1530s, provides corroborative evidence of the continued prevalence of sickness. In Panama City the "heat is so intense, and because the sun is so devilish, if a person takes it upon himself to walk under it, although for only a few hours, it will give to him such sicknesses that he will die, that exactly has happened to many." Furthermore, according to Cieza, "within the confines of this city there are few natives, because all have been consumed by the bad treatment that they receive from the Spaniards, and with the illnesses that they have had."[32] A decade later, Juan Cristóbal Calvete de Estrella vividly described conditions at Nombre de Dios and Panama at the time of La Gasca's 1546 passage: "These two towns are so infested, that of one hundred men who enter, if they remain in it for a

---

30 William S. Haubrich, *Medical Meanings. A Glossary of Word Origins* (New York: Harcourt Brace Jovanovich, 1984), p. 191. Mirko D. Grmek, *Diseases in The Ancient Greek World* (Baltimore: Johns Hopkins University Press, 1989), p. 131, notes that "Hippocratic *pleuritis* is actually most often either bacterial or viral pneumonia."

31 Teodoro Hampe Martínez, *Don Pedro de la Gasca: Su obra política en España y América* (Lima: Universidad Católica del Perú, 1989), pp. 86–87, 108, 111.

32 Pedro de Cieza de León, *Obras completas*, 3 vols. (Madrid: Consejo Superior de Investigaciones Científicas, 1984), 1:8–9.

month, there aren't twenty who are spared from sickness, and the majority of those who fall sick die." Thirty servants accompanied Pedro de la Gasca on the crossing, of these "two parts have died, even though they had all the things necessary to cure them with." After Gasca's mission in Peru was accomplished, he again passed through Nombre de Dios on his return voyage to Spain. The vicar of the settlement reported to him that "in the four months before he had arrived more than 600 had died in that town alone."[33] When Gasca and his group did depart from Nombre de Dios on their way to Havana, the members of the expedition were so ill that between the two ports, twenty-six corpses were tossed overboard, among them two shipmasters. The mortality was high even though this group had good medical supplies.

During the 1540s, substantial numbers of livestock (horses, mules, as well as pigs) were being imported into Peru from Spain, the Caribbean, and Nicaragua, for use in the military campaigns associated with the rebellion of Gonzalo Pizarro. Many horses and mules died; part of the cause was malnutrition on the long southward sea voyage from Panama to northern Peru. Yet disease as well as lack of fodder and drinking water led to deaths. Pedro de Cieza de León noted that Indians, llamas, and sheep were infected during the Andean version of the "great pestilence" that coincided with the civil wars of the conquerors.[34] Newson has pointed out that "it is known that during a plague epidemic these animals may also be attacked."[35] An epizootic in the Andes took two-thirds of the livestock between 1544 and 1545; some wild vicuñas and guanacos were also infected, although not as extensively. Dobyns found that Cuzco city records attest to an epizootic in the llama and sheep populations in 1546.[36] On the other hand, Alchon identifies the cause of Andean livestock deaths in the period as sheep pox, rather than rinderpest or anthrax.[37]

A severe epidemic was noted in the northern sector of South

---

33 Juan Cristóbal Calvete de Estrella, *Rebelión de Pizarro en el Perú y vida de don Pedro Gasca. Crónicas del Perú*, 5 vols. (Madrid: Biblioteca de Autores Españoles, 1964), 4:303.
34 Cieza de León, *Obras*, 1:134.
35 Linda A. Newson, "Old World Epidemics in Early Colonial Ecuador," in *Secret Judgments*, ed. Cook and Lovell, p. 95.
36 Dobyns, "Andean Epidemic History," p. 499.
37 Suzanne Austin Browne, "The Effects of Epidemic Disease in Colonial Ecuador" (Ph.D. diss., Durham: Duke University, 1984), p. 53.

America in the Quimbaya province of Colombia in 1546. Pedro de Cieza de León, who knew the region from close personal experience, wrote that "there came a general pestilence in all the kingdom of Peru, which began beyond Cuzco, and spread throughout all the land; countless people died. The illness consisted of a headache and a sudden very high fever, and then the pain passed from the head to the left ear, and the illness was so oppressive that the sick did not last more than two or three days."[38] According to Juan Friede, half the population of the Quimbaya succumbed to this epidemic.[39] Cieza's description of symptoms is one of the better contemporary accounts of any disease. Nevertheless, just as in central Mexico, there is considerable dispute over correct identification of the malady in the Andes. Cieza de León reported that mortality from the illness in the northern Andes was very high, as in Mexico, for it killed "countless people." The two most likely identifications are typhus and plague, probably pneumonic plague.

Just as the first smallpox and measles pandemics had a profound and lasting impact on the peoples of both Mesoamerica and the Andes, an impression that entered the popular mind, the terrifying disease episode of the mid-1540s led to the creation of legend. Pedro de Cieza de León reported that in the Quimbaya Province of Colombia a story was related that centered on the terrible epidemic of 1546. The setting was a half league from Cartago by the Consota River and a small lake, where residents prepared salt by evaporating spring water. Just before the epidemic erupted, local Indians were collecting salt and saw "a man, tall in stature, the abdomen torn open and the bowels and filth hanging out, and with two young children." As he approached some Indian women, he told them: "I assure you that I must kill all the women of the Christians and all the rest of you." Yet because it was still daylight, the native men and women to whom the apparition talked did not show any fear. "But they told the story, laughing among themselves when they returned to their homes." In a different village, that of Giraldo Gil Estopinan, people saw the same figure on horseback. "It swept as the wind through all the hills and mountains. Within a few days the pestilence and ear infections struck

---

38 Cieza de León, *Obras*, 1:36.
39 Woodrow Borah and Sherburne F. Cook, *Essays in Population History*, 3 vols. (Berkeley: University of California Press, 1971), 1:421; Juan Friede, *Los quimbayas bajo la dominación española. Estudio documental (1539–1810)* (Bogotá: Banco de la República, 1963), pp. 62–63.

in such a manner that the majority of the people of the province disappeared, and the Indian service women of the Spaniards died, and few or none remained. Furthermore there was such a feeling of dread that even the Spaniards themselves seemed terrified and frightened. Many Indian women and children claimed that they were able to see the presence of many Indians who had already died."[40] From Cieza's description, it seems that the sickness afflicted the European population also, and that mortality rates were ample to cause alarm. But the natives suffered an even higher death rate than the outsiders.

Chronicler Juan Calvete de Estrella reported what may have been another infection that afflicted Europeans most at the time. Along with the men on board the fleet that accompanied him was "verrugas, . . . so large, and even bigger that nits, in the noses, eyebrows and beards and they were of a pestilential humor between black and reddish. They caused pains and afterwards they peeled off, leaving one healthy." Medical historian Lastres wondered if it might have been "smallpox."[41] But given the context of the illness infecting mostly the Europeans, a more likely diagnosis is *Verruga peruana*, a form of Carrion's disease. Another account suggests "some reddish boils the texture of nuts, which form on the face, the nose and other places."[42] Some victims attempted to lance the boils, often with deadly results. The Italian traveler Girolamo Benzoni was infected in Puerto Viejo when he was there in 1546. He reported that practically all the Indians of the district came down with the infection. It was "of some verrugas that developed on the face and other parts of the body, the majority of which are the size of a nut. I also have suffered from them. They don't hurt; they are ugly and filled with blood. There is no other cure but to let them mature and cut them delicately with a thread."[43]

It is difficult to ascertain whether or not the series of epidemics of the mid-1540s spread to the hinterlands of the Americas. Dobyns suggested it did, but the evidence does not satisfy all investigators. Dobyns elsewhere argued that bubonic plague or typhus may have

---

40 Pedro de Cieza de León, *Crónica del Perú. Primera parte* (Lima: Pontificia Universidad Católica del Perú, 1986), p. 85.

41 Juan B. Lastres, *Historia de la medicina peruana*, 3 vols. (Lima: San Marcos, 1951), 2:76.

42 Linda A. Newson, *Life and Death in Early Colonial Ecuador* (Norman: University of Oklahoma Press, 1995), p. 146.

43 Girolamo Benzoni, *Historia del nuevo mundo* (Madrid: Alianza Editorial, 1989), p. 313.

struck the southeast of what was later the United States in the 1545–49 period. The Mesoamerican experience with the epidemic illness at the time is well documented, as we have seen. Dobyns, in joint research with Stoffle and Jones, considered that bubonic plague reached the Pueblo Indians in the Southwest in 1545 from original infections in Mexico. He further postulated that plague reached Florida by quick transmission by coastal canoes, slow overland passage, or relatively frequent shipwrecks along the south Florida coast. Although Dobyns can cite no specific reference in the Florida documentation, he suggests that its probability is "nearly certain" and argues that introduction of typhus came from a ship named the *Santa María de la Encina* that departed infested Veracruz on the Mexican coast in early 1549.[44]

The Florida expedition, under the religious leadership of Dominican Friar Luis Cáncer de Barbastro, was tragic from the start. Reaching landfall around Charlotte Harbor in May 1549, a party of four went ashore to enter into talks with the Calusa. One was an Indian woman, acting as interpreter, who carried the Christian name Magdalena. Friar Cáncer returned to the mother ship to secure more gifts, but when he returned to shore the group had disappeared. After several days spent sailing up and down in search of them, a Spaniard named Juan Muñoz paddled up with the news that the churchmen had been killed but that a sailor taken as a slave and Magdalena were alive still. Muñoz had been captured by Florida Indians ten years earlier during the Soto expedition and had managed to survive. Cáncer, in spite of warnings, put ashore and suffered martyrdom on 26 June. At this juncture, the ship and crew returned to New Spain. Low on water and provisions, the group limped back to their port of departure, "most of its crew was too ill with fever to work the craft." This "fever" in the view of Dobyns was probably typhus, for "most of the group was ill with fevers." According to Dobyns, the sailor, the Indian interpreter Magdalena, and the executed clergymen had taken the infected vector, the lice, ashore to plague the peninsula and its peoples. Dobyns also places mumps as possibly entering Florida from a core of infection in Mexico in 1550.[45]

---

44 Henry F. Dobyns, *Their Number Become Thinned: Native American Population Dynamics in Eastern North America* (Knoxville: University of Tennessee Press, 1983), pp. 264–65, 270.
45 Ibid., pp. 266–67.

WIDESPREAD INFLUENZA AND SMALLPOX, 1557–1564

McNeill stated that the influenza epidemic that raged in Europe between 1556 and 1560 "had serious demographic consequences on both
sides of the Atlantic."[46] It may even have been associated with an
outbreak of "coughing violence" noted in Japan in 1556, which caused
the deaths of many. Losses of life in Europe in general were high, and
in England one in five of its people died. Dobyns concurred that the
influenza outbreak that convulsed Spain in 1557 was pandemic in
much of Europe into the next year, and he pointed out that it could
easily have spread to the Americas aboard ships. It had fallen upon
Spanish forces fighting in North Africa in 1558 and had reached
Guatemala, according to Dobyns, by Easter 1559.[47] Indeed, it may
have spread through Guatemala before its introduction into central
Mexico.

Chronicler Francisco Vázquez wrote that a sickness characterized by
intense nosebleeds reached Guatemala in 1558. No cure could be
found, and a vast number of people succumbed. It was so severe that it
"almost destroyed the realm," according to Vázquez.[48] Officials of the
Audiencia of Guatemala reported on the conditions in the colony to
the monarch in Spain. In separate correspondence on 30 June 1560
and 7 February of the following year, they noted that "everyone is sick
and ridden with pestilence," and that "a very great number of Indians
have died." Colonial officials tried to assist the infirm Indians. The
symptoms provided in the *Annals of the Cakchiquels* are more explicit:
They include chills and fever, bloody discharge from the nose, followed by a "cough growing worse and worse," and a "severe sore
throat." There was a high rate of morbidity, with a massive number of
deaths. English versions of the text unfortunately vary, compounding
the difficulty of accurate diagnosis of the malady. Recinos and Goetz
translate "large and small sores broke out on them," but Brinton does
not mention these symptoms, nor do Spanish versions of the text.[49]

---

46 McNeill, *Plagues and Peoples*, p. 185.
47 Dobyns, "Andean Epidemic History," pp. 500–501; idem, *Their Number*, pp.
    269–70.
48 Lovell, "Disease in Early Colonial Guatemala," p. 73; Francisco Vázquez,
    Crónica de la provincia del santísimo nombre de Jesús de Guatemala (Guatemala:
    Sociedad de Geografía e Historia, 1937), 1:154.
49 Adrián Recinos and Delia Goetz, eds., *The Annals of the Cakchiquels* (Norman:
    University of Oklahoma Press, 1953), pp. 143–44.

Smallpox, measles, exanthematic typhus have all been suggested, and Lovell's conclusion that "the sickness might have been a combination of diseases" is valid. Because the Audiencia reports used the word *pestilence* and there was no direct mention of smallpox, measles, or typhus, I suggest that influenza should be added as another alternative diagnosis for what appears to be a compound epidemic series. The Cakchiquel text implies that it started in 1559 and was still rampant in mid-May 1562. Sickness continued into the next year, and drought, crop failure, and hunger prevailed. Lovell identified more localized disease outbreaks in Guatemala from about 1562 to 1564, at least for the district surrounding Chichicastenango. And smallpox visited the Cakchiquel in 1564.[50]

In the Mexican case, conditions in 1559–60 were propitious for a severe epidemic outbreak as a consequence of locust infestations that, coupled with frosts, led to crop failure and ultimately starvation. Disease followed, according to later information provided by Viceroy Martín Enríquez. On the Gulf Coast of what is today Mexico, according to the geographical report of Tuxtla, there was "vomiting of bile, the constriction or blockage of air passages, and death within six hours."[51] McBryde implicated influenza because of the symptoms of coughing and nosebleed, and he argued for linkage with the European pandemic.[52] Prem is skeptical and suggests diphtheria as a possibility, based on the Tuxtla symptoms. Mortality was not as severe as in the 1545–48 series in central Mexico; Prem thinks the Mexican experience may have been "a less than spectacular cluster of illnesses."[53] A more generalized epidemic outbreak took place in 1560, stretching from the Gulf Coast of Mexico into Guatemala. We do know that a relatively severe epidemic of measles afflicted some parts of Mexico in 1563–64, with mortality varying by location. Native American sources describe various symptoms, but a "sandy" or "blistery" rash over much of the body predominates, according to Prem. Some observers suggest smallpox rather than measles, and at least one mentions typhus (*tabardete*). Mortality in most places was relatively light. Chalco was an exception, for over half the native population there died within 18 months.[54]

50 Lovell, "Disease in Early Colonial Guatemala," pp. 72–75.
51 Prem, "Disease Outbreaks in Central Mexico," pp. 35–36.
52 Felix Webster McBryde, "Influenza in America during the Sixteenth Century (Guatemala: 1523, 1559–1562, 1576)," *Bulletin of the History of Medicine* 8(1940):296–302.
53 Prem, "Disease Outbreaks in Central Mexico," p. 37.   54 Ibid., pp. 37–38.

The Andean area in South America did not escape severe epidemic disease in the course of the late 1550s either. A significant smallpox outbreak in the northern Andes hit in 1558. It appears to have been introduced by infected slaves imported from Hispaniola by Bishop Juan de los Barrios of Santa Fé de Bogotá. Mortality was low for Europeans but high for native Americans. Symptoms were noted by Aguado (ca. 1581), who wrote that they were experiencing an out-break of highly contagious smallpox, "but those who came down with it swelled up and became damask-like, and were filled with worms and maggots that entered through their noses and mouths and other parts of the body . . . , and there were many deaths." One New Granada official lamented the loss of 40,000 Indians by September 1559. In October 1559 two officials wrote the king that "because of the sins of those of us who are in these lands, Our Lord has bestowed upon us a pestilence of smallpox as a punishment, such that many natives are missing."[55] An influenza outbreak probably coincided with the recurrence of smallpox.

In Ecuador both Europeans and native Americans were afflicted, with catarrh being prevalent. The compiler of the 1573 geographical report for the city of Quito reported that "in the year 1558 there occurred a general epidemic of smallpox among the natives. And other times some Spaniards and Indians died from a severe cough, which for the most part came at the beginning or end of summer months."[56] Alchon argues that the cough may have been a secondary infection that she links with the European influenza pandemic. "This coughing illness may have been an extension of the influenza pandemic which began in Europe in 1557 and would have attacked everyone, regardless of race or immunities to other diseases."[57] If so, the combination was lethal. Alchon concludes there was "high mortality . . . which led to further demographic decrease in Indian communities," and the effects lingered. The Indian village of Urinchillo, just to the south of Quito, was inspected in January 1559 for a tribute assessment. There was an abnormally small number of children between one and three, as well

55 Juan A. Villamarín and Judith E. Villamarín, "Epidemic Disease in the Sabana de Bogotá, 1536–1810," in Secret Judgments, ed. Cook and Lovell, pp. 118, 119.
56 Marcos Jiménez de la Espada, ed., Relaciones geográficas de Indias, Perú, 3 vols. (Madrid: Atlas, 1965), 2:205.
57 Suzanne Austin Alchon, Native Society and Disease in Colonial Ecuador (Cambridge: Cambridge University Press, 1991), pp. 55, 56.

as a relatively large percentage of orphans, widows, and widowers. This evidence, along with the list of the remaining ill provided by the officials, suggests the substantial local impact of the epidemic series. Alchon notes that "recent studies of influenza epidemics indicate that children, the elderly, pregnant women, and individuals suffering from other infections such as smallpox are especially likely to develop severe cases of the disease, which may eventually lead to viral pneumonia and death."[58] As late as 1562 in Cuenca, Ecuador, "still some or nearly all [Indians were] ill with smallpox." But it is unclear if "this was the tail end of the 1558 epidemic or a separate local outbreak."[59]

Farther northeast, and roughly on the border of present Colombia and Venezuela, the province of Pamplona (elevation 1,800–2,800 m) was first entered by Europeans around 1532. Conquest of the region began in earnest in 1539, and by the end of a decade settlement was firmly established. The effects of disease there are clearly visible from two population counts taken for tribute purposes. Pamplona was counted in June 1559 (31,850) by Cristóbal Bueno, then in April 1560 (20,700) by inspector Tomás López. An epidemic of smallpox had devastated the native peoples of the province, taking about 35 percent of the people in less than nine months.[60]

Much of Brazil's long coastline was beset by epidemic disease during the same period. Villegagnon's colony of French Antarctica at Rio de Janeiro was hit by an illness in 1556. André Thevet, one of our best sources for the venture, wrote, "This contagious malady ran everywhere so strangely that several of us died of it, and an infinite number of savages."[61] Spending roughly a year at the colony, Jean de Léry wrote that people called *pages* cured the sick by sucking on the part of the body where the sickness was concentrated. He complained that "these quacks would have them believe that they are not only extracting their pain, but even prolonging their life."[62] In addition to the common fevers and illnesses, the Brazilians experienced *pian*. Jean de Léry concluded that this was "the most dangerous disease in the

---

58 Ibid., p. 39.
59 Newson, "Old World Epidemics," p. 97.
60 Borah and Cook, *Essays in Population History*, 1:422–29.
61 John Hemming, *Red Gold: the Conquest of Brazilian Indians, 1500–1760* (Cambridge, MA: Harvard University Press, 1978), p. 140; from André Thevet, *La Cosmographie universelle* (Paris, 1575).
62 Jean de Léry, *History of a Voyage to the Land of Brazil Otherwise Called America* (Berkeley: University of California Press, 1993), p. 172.

land of Brazil." Léry described the symptoms: "pustules as wide as a thumb, which spread over the entire body, even to the face, so that those who are spotted with it carry the marks of their turpitude and baseness all through their lives."[63] Léry, not aware of the actual mode of transmission of the disease, assumed that it was sexually passed and confused it with syphilis. *Pian*, or yaws, is caused by a spirochete, *Treponema partenue*, whereas syphilis is the result of infection with *Treponema pallida*. The infection can come by contact with the organism through broken skin, especially on the feet and legs, or sometimes through the bite of a dipthos (fly). Incubation is about twenty-eight days. Yaws is one of four treponemal diseases that inflict populations, along with pinta, epidemic, and endemic syphilis. It is especially prevalent in the tropics, producing lesions similar to those of syphilis, and as it progresses over the long term, it too affects bones and joints.[64]

Smallpox may have been prevalent in the Rio de la Plata as well as elsewhere in Spanish South America from 1558–69, according to Alden and Miller. "By 1558–1560 *variola major* of unknown provenance had reached the Rio de la Plata, where geographer Juan López de Velasco tells us that it accounted for the deaths of more than 100,000 non-Europeans."[65] By 1559 fevers and hemorrhaging were widespread along the Brazilian coast. Espirito Santo was hit, and the disease spread to Bahia along routes in the interior. It continued in Bahia until 1561, then reappeared in São Paulo. Child mortality was high. Many who came down with the ailment died from "coughing and mortal catarrh" in a matter of four or five days. Hemming found symptoms of pleurisy and bloody fluxes and "fevers that they say immediately attacked the hearts, and which quickly struck them down." He concludes that the malady was probably "haemorrhagic dysentery, combined with influenza or whooping cough."[66] Dean pointed out that in the month of February 1559 the city of Espírito

---

63 Ibid., pp. 172, 173.
64 Don R. Brothwell, "Yaws," in *The Cambridge History of Human Disease*, ed. Kenneth F. Kiple (Cambridge: Cambridge University Press, 1993), pp. 1096–1100.
65 Dauril Alden and Joseph C. Miller, "Out of Africa: The Slave Trade and the Transmission of Smallpox to Brazil, 1560–1831," *Journal of Interdisciplinary History* 18(1987):215; idem, "Unwanted Cargoes: The Origins and Dissemination of Smallpox via the Slave Trade from Africa to Brazil, c. 1560–1830," in *The African Exchange: Toward a Biological History of Black People*, ed. Kenneth F. Kiple (Durham: Duke University Press, 1988), pp. 42–43.
66 Hemming, *Red Gold*, pp. 141–42.

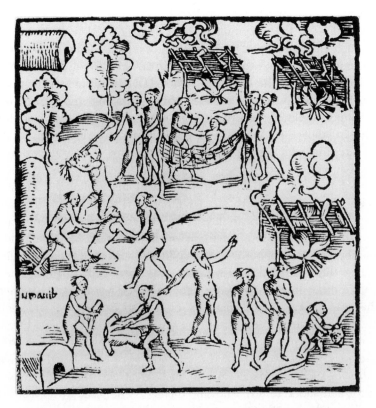

Figure 3.2. Hans Staden in Brazil, with sick visitor, ca. 1557.

Santo was hit by what appeared to be hemorrhagic dysentery and lung infections that moved northward along the coast and was carried by the natives trying to escape their infected homelands around Rio de Janeiro. "There it was reported that 600 died, of a population that may be estimated at no more than 3,000, including the countryside settlements, a loss of 20 percent."[67] The military campaigns of 1560–62 certainly had an impact on disease propagation. The transport of enemy captives further contributed to the spread of infection, and quickly at that.

More serious was the appearance of the plague in Lisbon in 1561; it

67 Warren Dean, "Las poblaciones indígenas del litoral brasileño de São Paulo a Río de Janeiro: Comercio, esclavitud, reducción y extinción," in *Población y mano de obra en América Latina*, ed. Nicolás Sánchez–Albornoz (Madrid: Alianza Editorial, 1985), p. 45.

may have been introduced into Brazil in conjunction with smallpox. Descriptions of the symptoms make it difficult to identify positively, although either smallpox or the plague, or a fatal combination of the two, might have been the culprits. Starting in 1561 in São Vicente, epidemics ravaged the coast until 1564. The island of Itaparica was devastated during three months in 1562. A second ship transported the illness to Ilhéus, and from there it was carried by sea, reaching Bahia in January of 1563. "The disease began with serious pains inside the intestines which made the liver and lungs rot. It then turned into pox that were so rotten and poisonous that the flesh fell off them in pieces full of evil-smelling beasties."[68] Dean argued that the series of illnesses included hemorrhagic dysentery, lung infections, and small-pox. Europeans and African slaves were also apparently afflicted. Jesuit Leonardo do Vale wrote a letter from Bahia on 12 May 1563 that describes the trials of both victims and those who tried to assist them. "When this last tribulation was past, and they wanted to raise their heads a little, another illness engulfed them, far worse than the other. This was a form of the smallpox or pox so loathesome and evil-smelling that none could stand the great stench that emerged from them. For this reason many died untended, consumed by the worms that grew in the wounds of the pox and were engendered in their bodies in such abundance and of such great size that they caused horror and shock to any who saw them."[69] The Jesuits who assisted the ill and dying had no time for sleep or the normal religious routine. Mortality was especially high for pregnant women. By the end, the uncounted numbers of dead had to be buried in mass graves, and "some were buried in dunghills and around the huts, but so badly that the pigs routed them up," wrote a contemporary.[70] Dean has suggested that the fear of the epidemic may have led the Amerindians to rise against the outsiders, hoping that if the foreigners were eliminated, the source of sickness would also be brought to a conclusion. "The terror provoked by the epidemic may have been a motive for the Tupiniquin uprising of 1562."[71]

Far north of Brazil, in the vast region of the southeastern part of the mainland of North America that the Spanish called La Florida, the influenza pandemic of 1559 coincides with the colonizing effort of Don Tristán de Luna y Arellano. As we have seen, the epidemic

68 Hemming, *Red Gold*, p. 142.   69 Ibid.
70 Ibid., p. 143.   71 Dean, "Poblaciones indígenas del litoral brasileño," p. 46.

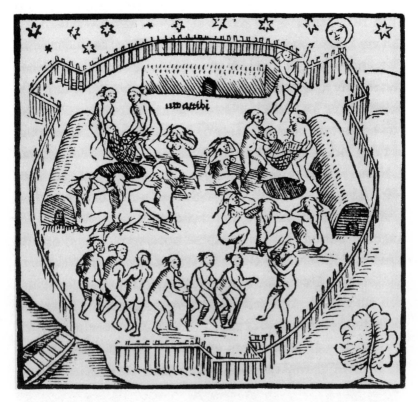

Figure 3.3. Hans Staden, burial practices among the Tupinamba, ca. 1557.

ravaged Europe in 1556, with English mortality being one in five. It hit Madrid in 1557, and Spanish forces in North Africa the next year. By Easter 1559 it was in Guatemala. The Luna group of thirteen ships with 1,500 men, women, children, African slaves, and some Indians, along with 240 horses, left the infected port of Veracruz on 11 June 1559. Their landfall on 14 August was at Ichuse, near modern Pensacola. A tropical storm destroyed most of their supplies, and the settlers suffered from hunger and disease. Some 800 stayed on at a place called Nanipacana, a village of eighty houses that the Indians had abandoned simultaneously with the arrival of the invaders.[72] In the Easter season of 1561, Angel de Villafañe arrived with supplies to replace Luna. Fewer than 300 people remained of the original settlement, and these

72 Dobyns, *Their Number*, pp. 269–70.

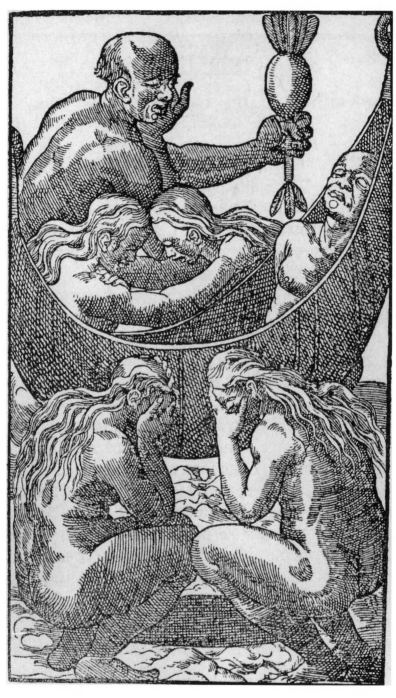

Figure 3.4. Brazilian shaman with sick natives, from Jean de Léry, *Histoire d'un voyage fait en la terre du Bresil* (1578), p. 174.

broken colonists, when offered the opportunity, opted to return to the mainland. Villafañe left a small force of fifty at Ichuse; these remained less than a year before the effort to colonize Florida was again abandoned.[73]

By the mid-1560s, final permanent European settlement of Florida was undertaken, the direct response to French encroachments and the Spanish decision to drive out the interlopers. Dobyns concluded that disease must have been present in the area between 22 June 1564 and 20 September 1565, a consequence of the large number of Europeans in a state of combat when the Spanish took the recently constructed Fort Caroline. Eyewitness Jacques Le Moyne depicted graphically the disease among the east coastal peoples, noting employment of hermaphrodites to provide nursing care for the ill. Timucuan treatments for illness were detailed by Le Moyne in a series of illustrations and accompanying text:

> They treat disease in the following way. They construct benches, which are as long and wide as can be seen in this picture, on which they place the sick face downwards or on their backs according to the kind of illness from which they are suffering. Then cutting the skin of the forehead with a very sharp small shell, they suck out the blood by mouth and spit it into some earthenware jar or into flasks made from a gourd. Women who are nursing male babies or who are pregnant come to drink this blood, especially that of any powerful youth, so that their milk may be made more nutritious and the boys brought up on it may turn out braver and more vigorous. For the others, who lie on their stomachs, they prepare fumigations by throwing some seeds over burning coals. For when the fumes are taken up through the mouth and nostrils they spread throughout the whole body and induce vomiting, or drive out and destroy the cause of the illness.[74]

The native Americans described by the French used some medical techniques that would have been familiar to European medical practitioners of the day. Bloodletting and purging were common practices used by Old World doctors to treat the sick.

---

73 Michael V. Gannon, *The Cross in the Sand: The Early Catholic Church in Florida, 1513–1870* (Gainesville: University of Florida Press, 1965), pp. 14–18.
74 Jacques Le Moyne de Morgues, *Brevis Narratio eorvm quae in Florida . . . 1564.* Text from plate 20 in Theodore de Bry's Frankfurt edition of 1591.

The Timucuas, as did other peoples in the Americas, used a variety of plants to cure disease. One was the sassafras tree. The prominent Seville doctor Nicolás Monardes was given a piece of sassafras by a Frenchman who had been in Florida and who extolled the curative properties of the infusion made with it. Monardes was skeptical at first "because much is said about these things of plants and herbs that are brought from foreign places, but little is known, unless a man tests it with care and diligence."[75] The Frenchman had told Monardes that when they arrived in Florida, "most had become sick, of various and grave illnesses." In Florida the Spanish also fell ill "from the poor food, drinking impure water, and sleeping in the open air, [and] most of them came down with continuous fevers, from which most became obstructed, and from the obstructions most became swollen."[76] The Spaniards were also instructed on the curative properties of the sassafras; indeed, Monardes describes sassafras as useful for a variety of ailments.

Tobacco was another medicinal plant used in Florida and elsewhere. Taking it from a pipe, "they [the natives] inhale the smoke so strongly, with the narrow part of the pipe placed in the mouth, that it comes out through their mouths and nostrils, and by this process it freely draws out the morbid fluids." Another participant in the French venture in Florida, René Goulaine de Laudonnière, wrote, "They have their priests, to whom they give great credit, because they are great magicians, great soothsayers, and callers upon devils. These priests serve them instead of physicians and surgeons. They carry always about with them a bag full of herbs and drugs to cure the sick who, for the most part, are sick of the pox." Doctor Monardes also described the use of tobacco and other plant products in the treatment of venereal disease: "Furthermore, they are extremely prone to venereal disease and for treating this too they have their remedies with which nature has supplied them."[77]

Compound Epidemics of 1576–1591

Epidemics that followed closely earlier ones appear to have done the most severe damage, and the 1576 to 1591 series was one of the

---

75 Nicolás Monardes, *Historia medicinal de las cosas que se traen de nuestras Indias occidentales que sirven en medicina* . . . [1574, facs. ed.] (Seville: Padilla Libros, 1988), p. 51v.

76 Ibid., p. 52r.

77 Ibid., p. 41; John R. Swanton, *Indians of the Southeastern United States* (Bulletin 137) (Washington, DC: Bureau of American Ethnology, 1946), p. 792.

deadliest. People already weakened by a bout with the first sicknesses were swept away quickly when they came down with a subsequent malady. As one approaches the end of the century, the documentary record improves. Indeed, the epidemic series of 1576–80 is one of the best documented for Mexico, in part because of the efforts of Spanish royal officials to comply with Philip II's order to compile the geographical descriptions (*relaciones geográficas*) for each province. According to Borah and Cook, the agricultural year 1575–76 had been marked by drought, crop failure, and famine.[78] The epidemic first appeared in August 1576, according to the Chimalpahin source, and by October the number of cases was declining. It appeared again early in 1577 and continued to April. The following year seemed to be free of disease, but illness resurfaced in 1579 in conjunction with other sicknesses.[79] Other similar patterns of flare-ups followed by abatements characterize the epidemic in central Mexico, with some areas being spared during one passage only to be hit in a subsequent onslaught. Such a pattern could easily be a consequence of the existence of two, even three or more different disease factors, thus complicating analysis of the series. Observers note that by the end of the half decade, most regions of Mexico and Guatemala had come under the influence of these deadly infections.

Mendieta identifies the sickness as typhus (*tabardillo*).[80] Symptoms included bleeding from all the body orifices. There was high mortality, and as we have noted, there may have been more than one disease element. Localized accounts in central Mexico labeled it *eztli toyacacpa quiz*, or "blood came from our noses." High fevers were usually followed by death within six to seven days. Especially detailed symptoms are to be found in the testimony given in the geographical report from Ocopetlayuca, which included "severe pain in the pit of the stomach," and is accompanied by a high fever in all parts of the body. "Death sets in after six or seven days . . . the sick who survive at this time become healthy. At the same time, there are cases of relapse with deadly consequences. No medicinal plant is effective against this disease."[81] Mortality was exceptionally high. On 26 October 1583 the archbishop of Mexico wrote the Crown to report the deaths of more than half of the native population. His estimate must have been based

78 Borah and Cook, *Essays in Population History*, 2:115.
79 Prem, "Disease Outbreaks in Central Mexico," p. 42.
80 Fray Jerónimo de Mendieta, *Historia eclesiástica de México*, 4 vols. (México: Editorial Salvador Chávez Hayhoe, 1945), 3:174.
81 Prem, "Disease Outbreaks in Central Mexico," pp. 39–40.

on a combination of sources: the death registers of Indian parishes, the fall in tribute revenues, new local population counts, as well as the impressionistic observations. The number of deaths in some cities was staggering; Torquemada simply estimated that in New Spain more than 2 million had fallen by the end of the epidemic. Blacks and some Spaniards also became ill from the disease. Reff traces the spread of the contagion northward into Zacatecas and along the west coastal road from Nayarit into Sinaloa. He found no record for the spread of this pandemic or of measles (1530–34) northward beyond the Tahue people.[82]

Many Guatemalan sources for the same years refer to smallpox, typhus, and colds. Martínez Durán adds plague (bubas), measles, and nosebleeds to the list.[83] Sicknesses arrived in Guatemala in 1576. On 13 March 1577, the royal accountant Eugenio de Salazar informed Philip II that "smallpox among the Indians has been contagious and widespread." Two days later, Lovell wrote, President of the Audiencia of Guatemala Pedro de Villalobos wrote to the monarch that "from Mexico has entered . . . a plague of smallpox and typhus, from which have died, and die daily still, a great number of Indians, especially young children." The epidemics continued into the following year. On 15 March 1578, Salazar again reported to the king, suggesting that because of the epidemics the Indians had been subjected to, they should be temporarily freed from tribute obligations. By then, lack of Indian laborers led to corn shortage. Other epidemics took place in Guatemala during this period: a 1585 grande enfermedad in Quetzaltenango, and in 1588 and 1590 disease outbreaks among the Cakchiquel. In 1588 the eruptive illness was deadly for children but not for elders. On 3 January 1590, there was an epidemic of coughs and fevers from which many people died. But, as Lovell points out, "the spatial impact of sickness could be highly localized, with disease occurring in some communities without necessarily reaching and infecting adjacent or surrounding ones." It is not clear when the series finally came to an end in Guatemala, but by 1582 the total impact on diminution of the native American population base was clear to all. That year the dean of Santiago de Guatemala cathedral, Pedro de Liévano, in explaining the disappearance of the Indians, testified, "What causes the Indians

---

82 Reff, Disease and Culture Change, p. 268.
83 Carlos Martínez Durán, Las ciencias médicas en Guatemala: origen y evolución (Guatemala: Tipografía Sánchez y De Guise, 1941), p. 71.

to die and to diminish in number are secret judgments of God beyond the reach of man. What this witness has observed during the time he has spent in these provinces is that from . . . Mexico have come three or four pestilences on account of which the country has been greatly depopulated."[84]

Disease was also a factor in reducing the number of Amerindian peoples to the south in Nicaragua during the same period. The best modern study of the situation in the region is by Newson, who found evidence that *romadizo*, or catarrh, hit Nicaragua in 1578. Both native Americans and Europeans were infected, but mortality was generally low for both groups. Pneumonic plague may have been present in Guatemala at the time, and a Honduran epidemic may have been a minor localized outbreak of the same disease. Newson also found documentation for an unidentified epidemic reported to have taken 300 lives in Nicaragua (1573) in only twenty days.[85]

In the Andes the 1570s were not as deadly for Amerindians as in Mesoamerica, but the following decade was. Speed of disease dissemination depends on a number of factors, of which population density is one important component. The higher the population density, the more rapid the spread of infectious community diseases. Native American depopulation in the years immediately after contact, and the dispersed settlement pattern found throughout most of the central Andes, led Spanish officials to attempt to congregate the Indians into villages. Clerics and bureaucrats had advocated concentration of people earlier, and Francisco Pizarro had even made a half-hearted attempt in the late 1530s. But instability and civil wars had prevented systematic application of the process through the mid-1550s. Beginning in the early 1570s, Viceroy Francisco de Toledo's resettlement program (*reducciones*) in the viceroyalty of Peru was designed to create a Christian utopia in the New World. Where earlier Andean residents had lived scattered in small communities of a few families, spread across the landscape, Toledo brought them together into villages of several thousand inhabitants, where they could be more closely watched, indoctrinated, and taxed. It was one of the most successful urban planning efforts in the Americas, and many of the towns established by the viceroy continue into the twentieth century. But unwit-

---

84 Lovell, "Disease in Early Colonial Guatemala," pp. 63, 76, 77–78, 82; Archivo General de Indias, Seville, Guatemala 10.

85 Newson, *Indian Survival in Nicaragua*, p. 247.

tingly, the viceroy established the conditions necessary for a new epidemic crisis by sharply increasing population density in an urban context. Quickly, Toledo's living utopia turned into a death trap for the Amerindian peoples of the Andes.

Within a decade after the *reducciones* had been established, a devastating series of epidemics passed through the Andes; it proved to be one of the most severe to hit the west coast of South America in the era and was just as disastrous as the one of central Mexico in the early 1580s. The duration and sharp impact of the 1585–91 crisis indicates that two, perhaps three or more, disease factors were operating. Indeed, sifting through the extensive evidence exposes the difficulty in dating the termination of one epidemic and the inception of another. The first seems to have afflicted Peru in 1585. According to Montesinos, smallpox and measles reached Cuzco in the form of a *peste universal* in 1585.[86] One city resident described the ailment as "high fevers with mumps" and claimed that thousands died in the city. The council of Huamanga (modern Ayacucho) closed the road with Cuzco to prevent the spread of the contagion, suggesting that the epidemic was moving westward.[87] What was described as *dolor de costado*, or pleurisy, was present at the same time, and the illness came with such force that those who were stricken suffered intensely. The epidemic recurred in Cuzco in 1590, with many Indian and creole victims. Father Barrasa in 1586 wrote about a smallpox epidemic in which young people were attacked with a merciless fury that reaped numerous victims. Native Americans were especially hard hit in this sweeping pandemic that stretched from Cartagena on the Gulf Coast of New Granada to Chile.[88] About 3,000 perished in Lima from the epidemic in 1586, mostly Indians, but many Blacks died too. As the rash healed, victims fell to "catarrh and cough," likely influenza or pneumonia, with the children and elderly the principal victims. Lima, with its population of approximately 14,262 in 1600, lost about 20 percent of its inhabitants to the 1586 onslaught. The city's Jesuits mourned six out of sixty of their own who died in the Lima house, so the death rate for the Jesuits was about half that of the population at large. In the Indian Hospital of Santa Ana fourteen to sixteen died

86 Lastres, *Historia de la medicina peruana*, 2:76–77.
87 Dobyns, "Andean Epidemic History," p. 501.
88 Lastres, *Historia de la medicina peruana*, 2:77.

each day for a period of two months; the consequence was that "an innumerable quantity of Indians died."[89]

Newson reports that an epidemic series, dated from 1586 to 1589, assaulted Quito and stripped away 4,000, especially children, within three months. It was characterized by "high fevers, smallpox and measles." Several epidemics swept Ecuador during the period, hence there is ample confusion over both accurate dating and reliable disease symptoms.[90] The first, according to Dobyns, was that coming from Cuzco. The second entered from the north. Jesuit José de Arriaga wrote to his superiors in 1590 that the sickness "first appeared in Cartagena . . . later passed to Quito and neighboring places as I have related in my previous letter. Later it spread not only to Lima, but also to Cuzco, Potosí and to all the southern part of the Kingdom of Peru."[91]

Andean South America was probably infected through the port and slave center of Cartagena de Indias, just as had happened in the 1558 Colombian epidemic outbreak. Old World disease could have been introduced in the normal course of the human trade, or it might have been the result of infections carried by the crew of the expedition of Sir Francis Drake. Drake had departed from Plymouth, England, on 14 September 1585, with about 2,300 men. The fleet stopped on 17 November at the port of Santiago in the Portuguese Cape Verde Islands. The residents of the town fled, and the English stole anything of value they could lay hands on. Unfortunately, they carried away far more than they realized. "There was adjoining to their greatest church an hospital, with as brave rooms in it, and in as goodly order as any man can devise; we found about 20 sick persons, all negroes, lying of very foul and frightful diseases. In the hospital we took all the bells out of the steeple and brought them away with us." They took more than church bells; they took the peal of death, for on 1 December, two days after leaving the islands, disease flared among the crew with a vengeance. Victims broke out with a "rash of small spots" and suffered high fever. Drake stopped at Dominica, traded with Indians, sailed on and attacked the Spanish city of Santo Domingo, then continued and

89 Dobyns, "Andean Epidemic History," pp. 501–502; José Toribio Polo, "Apuntes sobre las epidemias del Perú," *Revista Histórica* 5(1913):50–109; Lastres, *Historia de la medicina peruana*, 2:77.
90 Newson, "Old World Epidemics," pp. 97–98.
91 Dobyns, "Andean Epidemic History," p. 503.

took the port of Cartagena, occupying it for six weeks in early 1586. The attacking force in mid-March 1586 consisted of about 1,000 men. Continuing to be plagued by disease, Drake's forces passed sickness on to the permanent residents, who suffered greatly from its effects. Weakened by the disease, the English gave up and headed home, but they may have also transferred disease to St. Augustine. By the time the fleet set sail for the return to England, 750 men had perished, three-quarters of them from the fever taken in the Cape Verde Islands. Dobyns believes that the Drake group suffered from a vectored disease; because Europeans suffered too, it was not measles or smallpox but more likely typhus. Had it been bubonic plague, it would have probably been diagnosed accurately, for Spanish physicians had seen the plague all too frequently in Europe in the sixteenth century and could easily identify it.[92]

Alchon records the initial appearance of disease in Quito in or following 1585, and then chronicles the 1587 Quito outbreak in detail. In February 1587, the native American confraternity of the Holy Cross was so destitute that it was forced to petition the Audiencia to provide funds to help cure and bury those stricken by the disease. First noticed in July 1587, the epidemic continued for nine seemingly interminable months. A contemporary reported that 4,000 died during a brief three months; many victims were children.[93] According to the geographical report, the elements were "typhus, smallpox and measles . . . innumerable people, creoles, men and women, children and Indians" died.[94] The epidemic lingered in the Ecuadorian highlands well into 1590. Before the series subsided in 1591, "they left behind a trail of death and destruction unsurpassed by even the 1558 outbreak. In fact, the sharpest drop in Quito's native American population during the sixteenth century, at least as far as is presently known, occurred between 1560 and 1590; the epidemics of 1585–91 were primarily responsible."[95]

The Colombian disease experience of 1588 is also well documented. Castellanos noted that the epidemic came by way of an infected

92 Dobyns, "Andean Epidemic History," p. 505; Alfred Crosby, *The Columbian Exchange. Biological and Cultural Consequences of 1492* (Westport, CT: Greenwood Press, 1972); David Beers Quinn, ed., *The Roanoke Voyages, 1584–1590*, 2 vols. (London: Hakluyt Society, 1955), 1:378.
93 Alchon, *Native Society and Disease*, p. 40.
94 Jiménez de la Espada, *Relaciones geográficas*, 3:70.
95 Suzanne Austin Browne, "Effects of Epidemic Disease," p. 56.

female slave who had been brought from Mariguita on the coast.[96] The infection was present in Cartagena in 1588 and spread quickly throughout Colombia. Castellanos reported especially high mortality for "boys, girls, youth." Almost all informants from Colombia indicate smallpox as the principal component. One contemporary said that the 1588 bout was "one of the most unfortunate that the natives have experienced." It took more than a third of the population, striking Spaniards as well as Indians.[97]

Bernabé Cobo, who was an eyewitness, reported that the 1588 series covered Popayán and Quito and entered Peru. He traced the source of infection to trade goods imported on ships. It afflicted the black population and caused a "monstrous ugliness in the faces and bodies." Women were especially vulnerable; spontaneous abortions were commonplace in those who were infected. "The fetuses were not expelled from the womb, and they died from the force and the rigor of the fire and torment." Purges and bloodlettings, among the most common cures at the time, were used to combat the contagion, and, if we are to believe Cobo, the condition of many Indians improved with the bleedings.[98]

On 21 March 1589, Peruvian Viceroy Fernando de Torres y Portugal, the Conde de Villar, wrote to Philip II that the epidemic of "smallpox and measles" had reached coastal Trujillo. He had established a commission to block, by quarantine, the southward drift of contagion and to assist those who fell ill. On April 19, he wrote that in "the epidemic of smallpox and measles that began to hit the province of Quito, and from which some people have begun to die, the natives are receiving particular injury . . ., following it is a pestilential typhus. . . . In the highland provinces there has arrived, at almost the same time, another sickness of cough and *romadizo* with fevers, from which in Potosí more than ten thousand Indians have sickened, as well as some Spaniards. Up until now there has not been noticeable harm either in Cuzco or Huancavelica." Physicians Hierónymo Enríquez and Francisco Franco Mendoza advised the viceroy to recommend the use of sugar, oil, honey, raisins, and meat to help block infection. The all too common practice of bleeding was also cited as a

96 Villamarín and Villamarín, "Sabana de Bogotá," pp. 119–21.
97 María del Carmen Borrego Plá, *Cartagena de Indias en el siglo XVI* (Seville: Escuela de Estudios Hispano-americanos, 1983), p. 406; Villamarín and Villamarín, "Sabana de Bogotá," pp. 119–122.
98 Lastres, *Historia de la medicina peruana*, 2:77.

useful tool to save those who were sick. The viceregal recommenda-
tion to burn the clothing of those who died was an important positive
step to slow the contagion. It was precisely what the Conde de Villar
had ordered in Seville at the beginning of the 1580s as an effort to
block passage of the plague. Nonetheless, also on 19 April, the viceroy
wrote that smallpox and measles already had done their damage in
Quito, where they had "destroyed and killed a great number of Indians." It had reached Cuenca, Paitá, and finally Trujillo. In spite of the
best efforts of the medical commission, the sickness reached Lima in
June 1589, and by the end of the year it struck Cuzco.[99]

The Jesuit Provincial in Lima described victims in frightful detail:
"Virulent pustules broke out on the entire body that deformed the
miserable sick persons to the point that they could not be recognized
except by name." Dobyns found that "the pustules obstructed nasal
passages and throats, impeding respiration and food ingestion, occa-
sioning some deaths from these complications. Many survivors lost
one or both eyes."[100] The symptoms described in Cuzco parallel those
of Lima. The epidemic arrived around mid-September, in spite of
cutting transportation across the Apurimac bridge, halting the flow of
wine into the city, and conducting many religious celebrations to ward
off the approaching pestilence. The author of a Cuzco annal reported
ulcerated lips, eyes, and throats, with "tumors, callous excrescences or
itchy scabs or very nasty pustules." It was virtually impossible to
prevent those afflicted from scratching themselves, and Cuzco's smallpox victims were marked with "monstrous ugliness in faces and bodies." It is little wonder that most of those with the disease fell into
profound depression.[101]

The epidemic series greatly devastated Arequipa, where it erupted
in 1589. Joralemon identifies the Arequipa outbreak as "a combination
of fulminating and malignant confluent (variola major) smallpox." He
noted that typical mortality in this combination is 30 percent. Infants
tended to be affected most by the disease: "as recently as 1885 the case
mortality for ages 0–4 was 60 percent."[102] The symptoms in adult cases

99 Dobyns, "Andean Epidemic History," p. 505; Alchon, Native Society and Dis-
    ease, pp. 41–43; Roberto Levillier, ed., Gobernantes del Perú. Cartas y papeles,
    siglo XVI, 14 vols. (Madrid: Sucesores de Rivadeneyra, 1925), 11:207–208.
100 Dobyns, "Andean Epidemic History," p. 507; and Polo, "Apuntes," p. 56.
101 Dobyns, "Andean Epidemic History," p. 508; Polo, "Apuntes," pp. 16–17.
102 Donald Joralemon, "New World Depopulation and the Case of Disease,"
    Journal of Anthropological Research 38(1982):121.

in general were described in detail by Dobyns: "The onset of the disease brought severe headaches and kidney pains. A few days later, patients became stupefied, then delirious, and ran naked through the streets shouting. Patients who broke out in a rash had a good chance to recover, reportedly, while those who did not break out seemed to have little chance. Ulcerated throat extinguished the lives of many patients. Fetuses died in the uterus. Even patients who broke out in a rash might lose chunks of flesh by too sudden movement."[103]

Viceroy Villar on 11 May 1589 wrote Philip II that the illness was becoming less virulent in Peru's north and apologized that he had been unable to send more reports on local conditions "because everyone is ill and those who are well are very busy curing them." The sickness was spreading and recently had reached Lima, but at the time the viceroy reported to the monarch there were still few deaths, and most of those who did succumb were Blacks and native Americans. "But the illness is so general that there is scarcely a person in the place who is not touched with it." By the middle of June, epidemic-related deaths in Lima had soared. On 13 June, the viceroy wrote the king that "catarrhal smallpox and measles" was worse in the capital. His description of disease susceptibility is informative: "People have died in this city, among them natives and Blacks and mulattos and Spaniards born here, and now it has spread to those from Castile." All became sick, and mortality affected all ages in this compound series. On 16 June the viceroy lamented that disease had again hit Trujillo with renewed fury and that many natives and "even Creoles and Spaniards died" from "catarrh and pleurisy."[104] Dobyns believes that influenza moved from Lima into Peru's north, following the disease that produced the symptoms of a rash. But in Lima the rash bearing the sickness followed influenza. By 28 June Viceroy Conde de Villar sent an inspector to the communities of Surco, Lati, and Luringancho to set up hospitals supplied with beds and well stocked with medicines; on 12 July he named a surgeon to cure the ill for a tenure of six months in San Juan de Matocana, San Gerónimo de Surco, and San Mateo de Guanchor.[105]

Mortality levels from the compound epidemics were as high as any previous ones, perhaps even higher, because during these years, not

103 Dobyns, "Andean Epidemic History," p. 507; Jiménez de la Espada, *Relaciones geográficas*, 3:70; Archivo General de Indias, Lima 32.
104 Levillier, *Gobernantes del Perú*, 11:221, 284, 285–86.
105 Dobyns, "Andean Epidemic History," p. 506; Polo, "Apuntes," pp. 58–62.

Table 3.1. *Aymaya males' age
at death from smallpox, 1590*

Cohort	Smallpox deaths
0–4	36
5–9	30
10–14	5
15–19	7
20–24	24
25–29	23
30–34	12
35–39	6
40–44	0
45–49	1
50–79	0
80+	3
1,800 est.	147

Source: Evans, "Death in Aymaya,"
p. 152.

one epidemic but two or three coincided. If one suffered from one disease and survived, then was infected by a subsequent disease, the body's forces were incapable of fighting successfully the second infection. In the border districts between the Audiencias of Lima and Quito, deaths were exceptionally high. Native chiefs of the Jaén and Yaguarsongo districts reported in 1591 that, especially in the smallpox series, it was well known that in the valley of Jaén and province only 1,000 of an original 30,000 Indians remained.[106]

The epidemic series afflicted highland Charcas, too. Thanks to some exceptionally well-preserved records, Evans was able to study in detail one native-American community, Aymaya, from 1583 to 1623, and estimate mortality levels. The normal number of annual burials among the Aymaya in the 1580s was in the twenties. In 1590 the number exploded to 194, slightly over 10 percent of the community's population, based on Evans's estimate of about 1,800 as the total population of the Aymaya on the eve of the epidemic. (See Table 3.1 and Figure 3.5.) Of these deaths, 147 were listed in the registers as

106 Alchon, *Native Society and Disease*, p. 42; Archivo General de Indias, Seville, Quito 23.

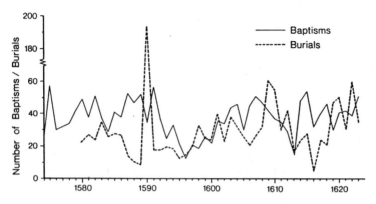

Figure 3.5. Baptisms and burials in Aymaya, 1574–1623, from Evans, "Death in Aymaya of Upper Peru," p. 148.

having been precipitated by smallpox. About 45 percent of deaths were of children under ten, again a reflection of the terrible impact of smallpox on the young. There were very few deaths among males over forty during the 1590 smallpox epidemic. This suggests that the cohort above the age of forty had experienced, or had at least been exposed to, one or more smallpox epidemics that had extended through the region in the decades before 1550.[107]

Most components of the series assailed the entire Andean region, ultimately flowing into Chile, where both Spaniards and Araucanian Indians were infected.[108] The 1585–91 epidemic series also invaded the upper Amazon basin and may have drifted downstream. We have noted the impact on Jaén, where the native population of 30,000 dropped to 1,000. Yaguarsongo and Pacamoros were hit hard. Between 1585–86 "pestilence" and "*enfermedades*" were reported in Loyola and Santiago de las Montañas. In Cangasa the population fell by more than a third. All these population centers have relatively easy access to the lower stretches of the montaña and the Amazon basin beyond. Unfortunately, measurement of the impact of disease in the Amazon basin is difficult, the consequence of inadequate documentation. The early descriptions of the expeditions of Francisco de Orellana (1541–42) and Pedro de Ursúa, and Lope de Aguirre (1560–61) make no

107 Brian Evans, "Death in Aymaya of Upper Peru," in *Secret Judgments*, ed. Cook and Lovell, pp. 142–58.
108 Dobyns, "Andean Epidemic History," p. 508.

Table 3.2. *Principal epidemic occurrences in America, 1519–1600*

Dates	Mesoamerica	Dates	Andean America
1519–21	Smallpox	1524–28	Smallpox
1531–34	Measles	1531–33	Measles
1545	Typhus, pulmonary plague	1546	Typhus, pulmonary plague
1550	Mumps		
1559–63	Measles, influenza, mumps, diphtheria	1557–62	Measles, influenza, smallpox
1576–80	Typhus, smallpox, measles, mumps	1585–91	Typhus, smallpox, measles
1595	Measles	1597	Measles

comment regarding poor health conditions in the places the explorers visited.

Foreign disease was inadvertently introduced to the peoples of the southeastern part of what became the United States, La Florida, many times during the course of the sixteenth century. The ill members of Sir Francis Drake's English fleet, as we have seen, carried sickness to Florida in 1586 on their way home from Cartagena in the Indies. Though much weakened by disease, the English stopped briefly, from 27 May to 2 June, and sacked the fortified port of St. Augustine on the Florida coast. According to the log of the *Primrose*, "The wilde people at first comminge of our men died verie fast and said amongst themselues, It was the Englisshe God that made them die so faste."[109] Four years later, another epidemic seemed to carry native victims to the grave. Royal accountant Bartolomé de Arguelles wrote to the Crown on 12 May 1591 that "this last year there was among them a mortality and many died, and also part of this cabildo and fortress was affected."[110] This epidemic, perhaps linked to the series that so seriously afflicted Mesoamerica and the Andean region, was probably separate from any sickness introduced by Drake.

Furthermore, epidemic disease struck Amerindians near the Raleigh colony on the coast of the Carolinas in 1587. Thomas Harriot reported

109 Quinn, *Roanoke Voyages*, 1:306.
110 University of Florida, P. K. Younge Collection, 33; Archivo General de Indias, Santo Domingo 229.

that after the English had toured hostile native-American settlements, "people began to die very fast, and in many in short space; in some townes about twentie, in some fourtie, in some sixtie, and in one sixe score." As Harriot said, this, in proportion to the size of the town, was substantial. "The disease also was so strange that they neither knew what it was, nor how to cure it; the like by report of the oldest men in the countrey never happened before, time out of mind."[111] Apparently no serious ill effects were experienced by the approximately 100 Englishmen there at the time.

During the sixteenth century, the native peoples of the Americas experienced one disaster after another. The Europeans brought not only their arms for conquest but also their plants and animals and their pathogens. It was not a single infection that came, but one, then another, a third, a fourth, and more. (See Table 3.2.) Just as the outsiders settled and became colonists, Old World diseases settled in, and some gradually became endemic. Taken together, the various epidemics resulted in a huge loss of life and led to relatively easy subjugation of an entire hemisphere. Of the several pandemics to sweep the Americas in the sixteenth century, three series stood out in the popular mind as watersheds. In Mesoamerica, Juan Bautista Pomar, who compiled the history of Tetzcoco, emphasized the three major killers: those in 1520, 1545, and 1576. For him the first plague was the most deadly. In the same vein, Diego Muñoz Camargo wrote in the 1580s of the impact of disease on Tlaxcala: "I say that the first [1520] ought to be the greatest because there were more people, and the second [1545] was also very great because the land was very full [of people], and this last one [1576] was not as great as the first two."[112] The sequence was similar in Andean America, although the third pandemic wave was especially devastating there because of the quick succession of highly mortal pathogens. Debilitated and convalescing peoples fell easy victims to fresh new infections.

111 Quinn, *Roanoke Voyages*, 1:378.
112 McCaa, "Spanish and Nahuatl Views," p. 428.

CHAPTER FOUR

Regional Outbreaks from the 1530s to Century's End

The mortality of the Indians was certainly fortunate for us; had it been otherwise we Christians might not have escaped alive.

Ulrich Schmidel, Paraguay–Paraná, 1530s–40s

The sorcerers delude them with a thousand follies and lies . . . preaching that we kill them with baptism, and proving this because many of them *do* die.

Francisco Pires, coastal Brazil, ca. 1552

During the course of the century following the tragic uniting of the disease pools of the Old World and the Americas in 1492, some of the foreign pathogens settled in and shifted from epidemic to endemic form. The original Greek terms illustrate the process; *epidemos*, or "visiting people," became *endemos*, or "living with people." In the seventeenth century, solely yellow fever, which required the proper conditions and a special carrier, would be a new arrival. It too would finally become endemic. Cholera did not appear in the Americas until the nineteenth century. The reason for its long delay is simple: The speed of transmission and the high mortality rate precluded cholera's transfer to the Americas aboard the slow galleons. Cholera's arrival in the New World was inevitable but only when sailing vessels were replaced by rapid steamships in the nineteenth century.

Not all regions were affected in the same way by the passage of a single epidemic. There were apt to be substantial variations, just as there were in Europe during the movement of the Black Death in the mid-fourteenth century. There, some cities (Florence, for example) lost 40 percent of their populations, whereas other places, such as Bohemia, escaped virtually unscathed by the initial European pandemic. Juan Friede rightly cautions that "when there were epidemics in Spanish America, these were neither general nor of identical consequences throughout the regions affected, contrary to what might be gathered from reading the various reports and chronicles of the colonial era."[1] Although, as we have seen, some clear-cut and well-documented examples of New World pandemics do exist, this does not permit us to ignore possibilities that many locally severe epidemics sputtered out and disappeared at various times and places in the Americas. From the 1530s onward, our disease chronology becomes more solidly established, at least in the case of the most severe outbreaks in well-settled districts. Pandemic occurrences continued during the course of the sixteenth century, often with very high mortality rates, especially for native Americans. These pandemics took place at approximate generational intervals, but by the mid-seventeenth century, several of the principal diseases, especially those that were arthropod vectored, settled down to an endemic-like, although still quite deadly, existence. This process can be well documented in central Mexico, a pattern that was repeated elsewhere in the New World.[2]

Some places were more frequently hit by disease than others, as the course of the epidemic history of the Americas clearly illustrates. Most observers mention the unhealthy nature of the isthmus of Panama. There were other places, often lowland districts with heavy rainfall and warm temperatures, that came to be characterized as unhealthy by Europeans and outsiders who complained loudly and frequently. Veracruz on Mexico's Gulf Coast, for example, quickly acquired a reputation as one of these. Founded in 1519 by Cortés, it was moved in 1521 because of sicknesses to a new and healthier location. And in 1524 Veracruz was moved for a second time. As early as 1531, when the city of Puebla was being established in the Mexican highlands, Veracruz was called the "tomb of the Spaniards." Friar Juan de Zumárraga wrote to the Council of the Indies in 1536 that 200 recent arrivals had been buried in Veracruz and that eight to nine continued to die daily. He suggested that July through September, a period during which the mosquito vectors are most active, were the worst months. The friar

1 Juan Friede, "Demographic Changes in the Mining Community of Muzo after the Plague of 1629," *Hispanic American Historical Review* 47(1967):341.
2 Hanns J. Prem, "Disease Outbreaks in Central Mexico during the Sixteenth Century," in *The Secret Judgments of God: Native Peoples and Old World Disease in Colonial Spanish America*, ed. Noble David Cook and W. George Lovell (Norman: University of Oklahoma Press, 1992), pp. 45–48.

argued that it would be advisable to cut off all communications with the outside world during this time. In 1556 an English traveler wrote that Veracruz was "very unhealthy and in my time many sailors and soldiers died of sicknesses that ruled there, and especially of those to which they were not acclimated."[3] Worst were the fevers, perhaps malarial, from which few escaped.

Recent research on the demographic collapse of Amerindian populations following contact with Old World inhabitants strongly points to an association between high mortality and coastal tropical environs.[4] Yet there are significant variations. The Gulf Coast region of Mexico, for example, suffered much more severe depopulation than did the Yucatán. And in the Yucatán there were discernible variations as well. By dividing the peninsula into subregions, Borah and Cook found that in the low bush country depopulation was less severe and recuperation came sooner. The large populations of the Yucatán of the high bush and tropical rainforest were by the mid-sixteenth century gone. Availability of rain and the conservation of water "has had a substantial role in conditioning the action of the factors unleashed by the Spaniards." On the central Veracruz coast in the high bush lands with heavy annual rainfall, we note a similar quick and massive fall in the numbers of Amerindians. By contrast, the low bush country, roughly the central Mexico plateau, underwent a less precipitous and slower population decline. "The comparison again points to the probable operation of disease as the major component among the lethal factors."[5] Fevers, perhaps malarial, are reported early in both native and European sources. Testimony referring to *quartanas* and *tercianas* is cause to suspect that malaria might have been present in humid and warm coastal sectors of the Americas.

There was a similar phenomenon along the coast of Colombia. In Peru, despite a more temperate, cool, and dry environment caused by the cold Humboldt current, coastal populations fell much more rapidly than highland populations in the century following Old World contact. Here, as in Mexico, there were regional variations. The Peruvian north coast, with a slightly warmer average temperature and higher humidity than coastal sectors to the south, may have suffered the

3 Miguel E. Bustamante, *La fiebre amarilla en México y su origen en América* (Mexico, 1958), pp. 27–28.
4 Woodrow Borah and Sherburne F. Cook, *Essays in Population History*, 3 vols. (Berkeley: University of California Press, 1971–79), 2:176.
5 Ibid., 2:179.

most severe early depopulation. The northern highlands, at a lower elevation and warmer temperature than the central and southern highlands, similarly experienced sharp depopulation. Perhaps primacy of contact and the size of non-American populations and density of settlement are factors as well as temperature and humidity levels. Certainly initial European activities in the Americas virtually everywhere were based along the coastline. The foreigners came by sea, they were reinforced by sea, and they departed by sea. Coastal port cities were the conduits for interior exploration and settlement. It is not then surprising that the greatest European–Amerindian contacts took place along the coasts and that disease spread there first before exploding into interior regions.[6]

MESOAMERICA

Prem's recent work on central Mexico is suggestive of patterns that likely hold elsewhere in Mesoamerica. In addition to the major pandemics of smallpox in the 1520s and the 1531–32 disease outbreaks, there were other severe but localized episodes. There was an epidemic of smallpox in 1538, according to the *Telleriano-Remensis Codex*, that resulted in "numerous deaths." Prem suggests that this may have been a regional appearance of smallpox, or that it may even have been the result of an error in recording. The 1545–48 series, well studied, was followed by mumps in 1550. Here the sources describe high fevers, swelling of the neck, and high mortality.[7] Prem warns that if mumps afflicted adult males, as it must have, then the long-term demographic consequences were assuredly severe, for fully one-third of mature males may become sterile as the result of mumps.[8] Several years later in central Mexico and the Yucatán, Borah and Cook report evidence for an epidemic in 1569–70 and drought and famine in 1571–72.[9] After the long series of the mid-1570s into the next decade, there were

---

6 Noble David Cook, *Demographic Collapse: Indian Peru, 1520–1620* (Cambridge: Cambridge University Press, 1981); Noble David Cook and George W. Lovell, "Unraveling the Web of Disease," in *Secret Judgments*, ed. Cook and Lovell, pp. 232–39.

7 Charles Gibson, *The Aztecs Under Spanish Rule: A History of the Indians of the Valley of Mexico, 1519–1810* (Stanford: Stanford University Press, 1964), p. 448.

8 Prem, "Disease Outbreaks in Central Mexico," p. 35.

9 Borah and Cook, *Essays in Population History*, 2:115.

other outbreaks. Both Friar Mendieta and Mexico City council records cite food shortages and higher than usual sickness and deaths in 1587; in the record for 9 September the term *cocoliztli* is used. Other sources mention the sickness but do not give the symptoms.[10] In 1595 there was another epidemic sequence in central Mexico. Mendieta reported three distinct disease factors: measles, typhus, and mumps.[11] Other sources for Mexico mention solely measles, although Prem considers that smallpox might have been prevalent too.[12]

Informants in the community of Coatepec, in the diocese of Mexico, also provided testimony to colonial officials in 1579 regarding health and disease. Village elders reported that when they were still pagan, before the arrival of the foreigners, they experienced various illnesses: fevers recurring on the third and fourth days, syphilis, bloody stools, infected eyes, and fevers. They treated and cured most patients with a variety of effective herbs and medicinal roots. But they bemoaned the fact that "after the Spaniards arrived other illnesses that they had not known occurred, such as smallpox, measles, pleurisy, typhus, influenza, mumps, hemorrhoids, and this pestilence that is now present that did not exist before." One of the native remedies was bloodletting, but instead of taking it from the arms as was common in Europe, they took it from the head or chest and abdomen, using a thin, sharp stone or viper fang. Mostly they used herbs and medicinal roots to try to effect cures. In the nearby village of Chimalhuacan, informants provided similar testimony on pre-Columbian sickness. Furthermore, they reported the arrival of new illnesses "such as measles, smallpox, typhus, and the sickness of *cocoliztle* that presently spreads." (See Table 4.1.)

Excellent testimony on health and disease was also extracted from the community of Tepuztlan in 1580. Before the arrival of the Europeans, the principal complaint was fevers, but "now, in the present time, a thousand varieties of sicknesses persecute them, such as: *matlaltotonque*, that is what we call 'tabardete,' they call it thusly because of the spots [*manchas*] that they discover on the body; and another that they call in their language *matlalcagua* that is the same as 'measles and bloody stools and bleeding from the nose.' " The witnesses complained that none of these were known before the coming of the Spaniards. A

10 Prem, "Disease Outbreaks in Central Mexico," p. 42.
11 Fray Jerónimo de Mendieta, *Historia eclesiástica de México*, 4 vols. (México: Editorial Salvador Chávez Hayhoe, 1945), 3:174.
12 Prem, "Disease Outbreaks in Central Mexico," p. 43.

Table 4.1. *Epidemics in central Mexico,*
1519–1600

Dates	Disease
1520–21	Smallpox
1531–32	Measles
1545–48	Typhus
1550	Mumps
1559	Typhus or pneumonic plague
1563–64	Measles
1566	Cocoliztli
1576–81	Typhus
1587–88	Cocoliztli
1590	Influenza
1592–93	Measles
1595–97	Measles, typhus, mumps

Source: Prem, "Disease Outbreaks in Central
Mexico," p. 47; and Whitmore, *Disease and
Death*, p. 53.

host of herbal cures were effected in Tepuztlan, many of them supposedly for *tabardete*. But regarding a possible cure for measles and bloody
stools, witnesses reported that "they have taken many herbs and they
have found none effective against them."[13]

Reff, with access to better records for northwestern New Spain after
1591, when the Jesuits were firmly in place, suggests that smallpox first
hit the area as an epidemic in 1593. Because sickness came after
baptism, the natives associated smallpox with the arrival of the Black
Robes and the rites of the church, as was the case in coastal Brazil and
elsewhere. Child mortality was very high among the mission Indians.
In Sinaloa, Father Gonzalo de Tapia complained that two out of three
children he baptized during the bout of 1593 died.[14]

By systematic search in archives in both Spain and Guatemala,

13 Alfredo López Austin, *Textos de medicina nahuatl* (México: UNAM, 1975), pp.
131–32.
14 Daniel T. Reff, "Contact Shock in Northwestern New Spain, 1518–1764," in
Disease and Demography in the Americas, ed. John W. Verano and Douglas H.
Ubelaker (Washington, DC: Smithsonian Institution Press, 1992), pp. 268,
270.

Table 4.2. *Major Guatemalan epidemics, 1519–1600*

Dates	Disease
1519–21	Smallpox, measles, influenza or pulmonary plague
1533	Smallpox, measles
1545–48	*Gucumatz*, typhus, pulmonary plague (?)
1558–63	Smallpox, measles, typhus
1576–78	Smallpox, measles, *tabardete* (typhus), *bubas* (bubonic plague?)

Source: Lovell, "Disease in Early Colonial Guatemala," p. 59.

Lovell located a number of important regional, or localized, epidemic outbreaks apart from the pandemics that assaulted the realm. Around 1555 there were "sicknesses and deaths" in Zamayeque. During the late 1550s and early 1560s, mortality was high, and the illness disrupted the normal production and supply of foodstuffs, which caused starvation. The compiler of the *Annals of the Cakchiquels* poignantly wrote that "in the sixth month after the arrival of the Lord President in Pangan [Juan Núñez de Valdecho, 1560], the plague which had lashed the people long ago began here. . . . Now the people were overcome by intense cold and fever, blood came out of their noses, then came a cough growing worse and worse, the neck was twisted, and small and large sores broke out on them. The disease attacked everyone here." But more than the description of the symptoms is the agony suffered by the people, including the record-keeper. "On the Day of the Circumcision [1 January 1560], a Monday, while I was writing, I was attacked by the epidemic." Mortality was high. "Seven days after Christmas the epidemic broke out. Truly it was impossible to count the number of men, women, and children who died this year. My mother, my father, my younger brother, and my sister, all died. Everyone suffered nosebleeds. Sickness and death were still rampant at the end of the sixty-third year after the revolution [18 May 1562]."[15] (See Table 4.2.)

15 George W. Lovell, "Disease and Depopulation in Early Colonial Guatemala," in *Secret Judgments,* ed. Cook and Lovell, pp. 75–76; Adrián Recinos and Delia Goetz, eds. *Annals of the Cakchiquels* (Norman: University of Oklahoma Press, 1953), pp. 143–44.

Regional Outbreaks in the Andes

Channels of epidemic penetration of South America were located at coastal enclaves around strategic port cities. The Spanish, by the 1530s, had established towns at Santa María la Antigua del Darién (1510) near the Panama–Colombia border, Panama (1517), Cumaná (1516), and Coro (1527) in what became Venezuela, Santa Marta (1525) and Cartagena (1533) on the north coast of what is today Colombia, Guayaquil (1537) in Ecuador, and Lima (1535; Callao was the nearby port) in Peru. We have already noted the Federmann report of a killer disease that had passed through the spur of the Andes jutting into Venezuela in the area near Coro several years before his men traversed the district in 1530–31. In the northern part of Andean South America, as one moves into today's Colombia, the early disease chronology is difficult to establish reliably. The broken terrain, the heavy rainfall, and the bellicose inhabitants made the Europeans cautious in their initial attempts at reconnaissance. The first significant recorded contact with the Chibcha in the Sabana de Bogotá did not take place until 1537, and it is possible that at least two major disease outbreaks (smallpox in the 1520s, and measles and influenza in the early 1530s) preceded this contact. Pedro de Cieza de León provides the earliest useful notice of epidemic disease in what is now southern Colombia, with a "pestilence in the houses" in Popayán in 1539.[16] It was said to have coincided with famine and to have taken 100,000 lives. The early seventeenth century chronicler Antonio de Herrera gave the epidemic the vague label of *peste* and reported that it caused the sudden death of those who contracted it. He argued that it killed 100,000 but that another 50,000 died from hunger or cannibalism.[17] Juan Friede claimed that measles and smallpox struck Cartagena on the north coast of Colombia at the same time.[18]

Far to the south, in the city of Cuzco, Diego de Almagro was ill in 1538, suffering from fevers and severe pains. "It was said that he was

---

16 Pedro de Cieza de León, *Obras completas*, 3 vols. (Madrid: Consejo Superior de Investigaciones Científicas, 1984), 1:127.

17 Antonio de Herrera y Tordesillas, *Historia general de los hechos de los castellanos en las islas y tierra firme del mar océano*, 17 vols. (Madrid: Real Academia de la Historia, 1934), Dec. 6, lib. 6, cap. 1:12.

18 Juan Friede, ed., *Documentos inéditos para la historia de Colombia*, 10 vols. (Bogotá: Academia Colombiana de Historia, 1955–60), 5:148.

covered with the pox [*bubas*] and was very thin."[19] Captain Diego de Almagro spent his last days, after his defeat at the Battle of Salinas by the Pizarro forces, in agony. His body was filled with boils (*bubas*); the symptoms suggest syphilis. Yet Almargo did not die from the sickness he was suffering from; instead, he was executed by the Pizarrists. Almagro, as did many other Europeans engaged in the exploration and pacification of Andean America, mentioned syphilis-like lesions, but these may have been caused by other illnesses.

Most foreigners were convinced that syphilis and other ailments could be cured by the sarsaparilla plant. Pedro de Cieza de León described it in excellent detail, noting that fine specimens could be found along the Pacific Coast of South America at Puná Island and Guayaquil. "The roots of this herb are useful for many sicknesses, and above all for the illness of pox [syphilis], and the pains given to men by this pestiferous illness." Cieza de León noted that many of his companions had become infected: "Ultimately, many were inflamed, and others ulcerated, and they returned to their homes cured." Later, when Cieza de León was traveling in the central Peruvian highlands near Vilcas, he admitted that one of his slaves was infected, "by being ill with certain ulcers which she had in her lower parts." He reported that in exchange for a llama "that I gave to some Indians, I saw that they carried some herbs and took out a yellow flower, and toasted it over a flame to make it into a powder, and with two or three applications as an ointment she was left cured."[20]

There is one reference to a general epidemic in Peru in the early 1540s, although it seems to have afflicted only a section near the city of Arequipa. On 22 January 1540, Francisco Pizarro had granted an encomienda of 800 tributaries to one of his loyal followers, Juan de la Torre. These Indians, in Condesuyos, were counted and taxed promptly, but a recount had to be made shortly afterward "because of the Indians who died in the general epidemic."[21]

The following two decades witnessed few major epidemics in Ecuador. A localized outbreak of smallpox may have occurred in Almaguer in the south highlands of Colombia in 1566, perhaps reaching eastern parts of Colombia in 1568–69. A severe bout of smallpox was reported in December 1566, and another in March 1571, in Pasto. Indeed, smallpox and measles may have settled down in endemic form. In

19 Ibid., 5:433.   20 Cieza de León, *Obras completas*, 1:78–79, 135.
21 Archivo General de Indias, Seville, Justicia 432.

1582, for example, in Cuenca, according to testimony of Hernando Pablos in his geographical description of the province, the two diseases were appearing "according to their seasons." In fact, a particularly severe smallpox epidemic outbreak hit the Cuenca region that very year.[22] (See Map 4.1.)

PERIPHERY: LA PLATA TO TIERRA DEL FUEGO

References to the relationship between disease and New World conquest in peripheral regions outside the circum-Caribbean and the Mesoamerican and Andean heartlands abound, albeit they are scattered. Indeed, in the case of coastal Brazil and the northeast of North America, the records become relatively good, especially after the middle of the sixteenth century. These were lands peripheral to Spanish interest, for the Castilians tended to concentrate on the areas that were most productive of riches or the outposts that were too significant in strategic location to allow them to fall into someone else's hands. The Dutch, the English, and the French all became involved in American exploration and discovery, trade, and ultimately settlement. Some of the accounts of their endeavors provide excellent information on the disease climate. In both the Amazon basin of Brazil and its coast, and the St. Lawrence to the Great Lakes region of Canada, the detailed Jesuit records allow for a more complete disease chronology to be established.

The discovery of the icy windswept rocky land of Tierra del Fuego at the southern tip of the great American land mass came as the logical consequence of the efforts of Christopher Columbus to reach the Orient by sailing directly westward. Just as there were many attempts by various explorers to find a northwest passage to the East in the last half of the sixteenth century, so too, after reconnaissance of the eastern coasts of America, exploration was directed to the south. The most spectacular voyage and the first to prove successful was that of Ferdinand Magellan and his companions. Yet Magellan had been beaten to the southeast coast of South America by Juan de Solís, who

---

22 Marcos Jiménez de la Espada, ed., *Relaciones geográficas de Indias: Perú*, 3 vols. (Madrid: Atlas, 1965), 2:266; Linda A. Newson, *Life and Death in Early Colonial Ecuador* (Norman: University of Oklahoma Press, 1995); Luis F. Calero, *Chiefdoms Under Siege. Spain's Rule and Native Adaptation in the Southern Colombian Andes, 1535–1700* (Albuquerque: University of New Mexico Press, 1997), p. 86.

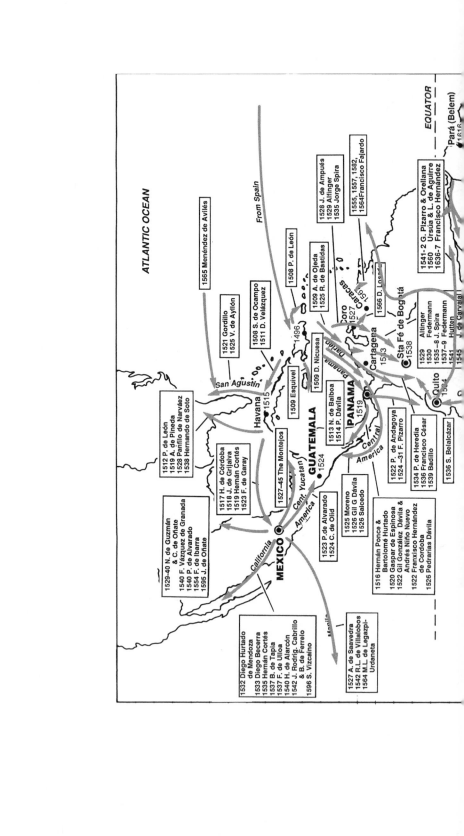

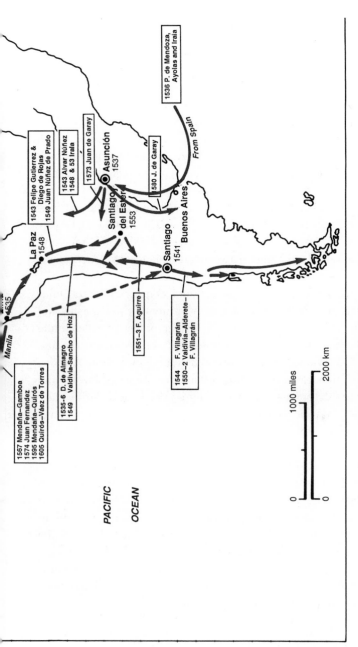

Map 4.1. Spanish voyages of exploration to mid-seventeenth century.

discovered the Rio de la Plata estuary in 1516. Magellan left Spain in 1519, stopping at Rio de Janeiro to pick up a mestizo son of one of his crewmembers; the boy's mother was a Tupinamba. In addition to the profits to be made in brazilwood and parrots, the free-spirited and sexually uninhibited Tupinamba women proved to be alluring and irresistible to European sailors. In all, about ten known Spanish expeditions touched the Brazilian coast before 1555, some associated with a search for a southwesterly passage to the Orient, some looking for an easy Atlantic route to precious metals in the Andean mountains, and others wanting arable lands in the Rio de la Plata region. Sebastian Cabot, for example, made an unsuccessful attempt to colonize the Rio de la Plata area in 1526. In 1528 he sailed up the Plata and encountered a large party of unintimidated Evueví Indians. Many people were involved in contacts in the region between 1500 and 1550, and substantial biological exchange between Europeans and Amerindians took place.[23]

Contacts with the upper Rio de la Plata continued in the mid-1530s. In 1536 Juan de Ayolas took Cabot's route up the Paraguay and Paraná rivers with a substantial force. Under orders of Adelantado Pedro de Mendoza, he journeyed far north and west of Asunción, and with about 300 Evueví guides continued inland into what is today Bolivia, where they came into contact with the Caracues. Ayolas and his men (some 200 Spaniards) were killed by the Evueví during their return to the Atlantic coast.[24] The Spanish in 1542 sent a large expeditionary force to retaliate, and a number of warriors were captured and burned at the stake under orders of Alvar Núñez Cabeza de Vaca. Ulrich Schmidel provides one of the more complete early accounts of European actions in the area and includes some information on disease. Schmidel, a native of Straubing on the Danube River in Lower Bavaria, traveled and fought for many years (ca. 1534–54) in the lands of the Paraguay–Paraná basin. He had shipped out of the port of Seville with the fleet of Captain-General Pedro de Mendoza. For almost two decades he participated in the exploration and subjugation of native American groups from the Pampas into the Gran Chaco and beyond to the edge of territory claimed by Portugal. He traveled

23 Warren Dean, "Indigenous Populations of the São Paulo–Rio de Janeiro Coast: Trade, Aldeamento, Slavery and Extinction," *Revista Histórica* (São Paulo) 117(1984):10–11.
24 Barbara J. Ganson, "The Evueví of Paraguay: Adaptive Strategies and Responses to Colonialism, 1528–1811," *The Americas* 45(1989):470.

for a time with Alvar Núñez Cabeza de Vaca and later fought under Captain-General Domingo Martínez de Irala. He finally returned to Germany in 1554, where he composed his chronicle in 1562–65 (published in 1567).[25]

During the infamous Cabeza de Vaca entrada, Schmidel and other explorers voyaged upriver from the young settlement of Asunción in search of the Amazon. Passing many ethnic units, they ultimately reached the "nation" of the Orthueses during the rainy season, having spent many days plodding with great difficulty over flooded terrain. Schmidel admired the size of the principal Orthueses settlement: "There were so many people, that in all the Indies I have not seen another settlement as large, nor so many Indians together, as in this one which was very long and wide." Schmidel acknowledged that "the mortality of the Indians was certainly fortunate for us; had it been otherwise we Christians might not have escaped alive." He ventured that deaths were largely due to famine, because "the locusts had eaten and devastated the carob trees twice, and they had nothing left to eat." According to Schmidel, many Spaniards were also ill at the time, and he blamed it on the water. Late in 1543 or early 1544, Cabeza de Vaca was "ill with fever and confined in his house for 14 days when they returned to Asunción." Schmidel complained that "at that time I was ill with dropsy, and very weak, as a result of the expedition to the Orthueses, when we had to go such a long time through water; furthermore, we suffered great want and hunger. In this voyage eighty became ill, of which only thirty escaped alive."[26]

Certainly a communications link from the Andean highlands into the Paraguayan watershed, although still imperfect, was being established in the decade of the 1540s. Pedro de la Gasca had sent letters to the Rio de la Plata settlement to ensure that Gonzalo Pizarro's supporters would not find refuge there and later challenge royal authority. Captain-General Domingo Martínez de Irala sent four commissioners to report to Gasca in Peru, traveling first to Potosí, then Cuzco, and finally Lima. The trip to Peru took a month and a half.[27] The establishment of the Paraguayan encomienda system in 1556 by Governor Domingo Martínez de Irala resulted in increasing contacts between native Americans and Europeans; 20,000 natives were distrib-

---

25 Ulrich Schmidel, *Relatos de la conquista del Rio de la Plata y Paraguay 1534–1554* (Madrid: Alianza Editorial, 1986).
26 Ibid., pp. 70–71, 74–75, 76.   27 Ibid., pp. 96–97.

uted to 320 colonists. The personal service requirement, so pervasive among the Guaraní, was to accentuate contacts, and widespread trade facilitated the spread of disease. In the brief period from 1571 to 1581, major new settlements in the region were established, and a number of important towns were founded: Corrientes, Santa Fé, Santa Cruz de la Sierra, Mendoza, and the second Buenos Aires. In the sector near Asunción, Franciscan Friar Luis de Bolaños set up eighteen missions in the next dozen years (1581–93).[28]

Coastal Brazil

The disease chronology for the coast of Brazil is understood in its basic lines, although knowledge of what happened in the Amazon basin remains sketchy. With the growth of the slave trade that was so important for the development of the coastal sugar industry, the disease cycle of Brazil came into a close relationship with that of coastal West Africa. The Portuguese colonists attempted to control the spread of disease by inspection of slave cargoes and applied quarantine when necessary, but these methods were only partly successful. Some of the major epidemics entered Brazil in spite of quarantine and quickly swept beyond the confines of Portuguese territory into areas under the domination of Spain.

The eastern coast of Brazil was discovered by Portuguese explorers in 1500 as they voyaged to the Orient via the route of the African Cape of Good Hope. The north coast of the continent of South America was touched by Columbus during his third voyage around 1499. The Italian Amerigo Vespucci, whose name was placed on the map of the continent by German cartographer Martin Waldesee-müller, acted as Columbus's pilot. It has been estimated that between 1500 and 1550 at least 330 ships from several nations made contact with the Tupinamba section of the Brazilian coast, with 10,000 Europeans potentially involved in the biological exchange.[29] In the coastal strip of Brazil populated by the Tupinamba, there were several instances of early contact. Gonçalo Coelho's expedition reached the area in 1501, examining the territory between Cape Frio and the Guanabara Bay and securing some brazilwood; Vespucci also participated in this trip. There may have been another 1501 expedition. The

28 Ganson, "The Evueví of Paraguay," p. 471.
29 Dean, "Indigenous Populations," p. 10.

Table 4.3. *Epidemics along the Brazilian coast,*
1500–1600

Dates	Epidemic
1527(?)	Fevers
1552	
1554	Fevers and bloody fluxes
1556	Contagious malady
1559–61	Fevers and hemorrhaging, mortal catarrh, hemorrhagic dysentery with influenza, whooping cough
1562–63	Smallpox, or plague
1565	Smallpox (in Espírito Santo)
1575	Smallpox and measles
1597	Smallpox

Sources: See citations in text.

1502–3 map of Nicolau de Caveiro details that part of the coast well and may be based on information collected before Coelho's reconnaissance of 1501. In 1504 a Frenchman, Paulmier de Gonneville, touched the Tupinamba coast. He claimed that others had sailed out of the port of Honfleur "for several years," prior to the Portuguese announcement of their discovery of Brazil in 1500. Hence, we must conclude that European-American contacts took place early along Brazil's coast, just as was the case in the far northeast part of North America on the Newfoundland fishing banks. By 1519 an average of two Portuguese trading ships per year were anchoring off the Tupinamba coast. French involvement intensified after 1519, with about six ships each year trading at Cape Frio. There were also English ships as well as others. By 1555 at least ten Spanish expeditions had touched the Tupinamba coast. Such continuous and substantial contact contributed to the transfer of pathogens. (See Table 4.3.)

While Sebastian Cabot's fleet was harbored at Lagoa dos Patos in 1527, many of the men on board died of a fever. Both criminals and the ill were often abandoned along the Brazilian coast by their compatriots. For example, Englishman Anthony Knivet and others stricken in the Cavendish expedition of 1591 were put ashore. The log of Pero Lópes de Sousa's voyage of 1531, according to Dean, "provides dramatic evidence of the terror induced by epidemics on shipboard."[30] Naturally the Europeans thought it humane to land their ill compatriots where they might be cured, but any European disease they carried would thus be introduced quickly into the local populations.

It is not until the first permanent Portuguese settlements were established along the Atlantic coast that we begin to have available reliable information on the peoples of the area. From the 1550s onward, the coastal strip was swept by wave after wave of epidemic disease. Friar Francisco Pires wrote in 1552 to his Jesuit superiors that disease had ravaged the first converts near Bahia. "Almost none of these has survived," he complained. The situation became so bad that shamans were able to convince the Tupi peoples that the Jesuits were the cause of death and destruction. "The heathen fled from the Fathers and Brothers as if from death: they abandoned their houses and fled into the forest. Others burned pepper to stop death from entering their houses." Missionaries lamented that "The sorcerers delude them with a thousand follies and lies . . . preaching that we kill them with baptism, and proving this because many of them *do* die."[31]

An epidemic broke out in São Paulo in 1554. The symptoms reported were violent fevers and bloody fluxes. An eyewitness reported that the illness "struck with such violence that as soon as it appeared it laid them low, unconscious, and within three or four days it carried them to the grave."[32] It might have been pneumonic plague. In all likelihood this is the epidemic described by the German Hans Staden, who was captured and held by the Tupinamba. Staden sailed initially to the New World under the Portuguese flag in 1547. The fleet had landed in the Madeiras, touched the African coast, then sailed to the eastern tip of Brazil at Olinda, then finally returned to Portugal in October 1548. The second trip was out of southern Spain in 1550, as part of a large fleet. According to Staden's account, they left Sanlúcar, landed in the Canaries at Palma to purchase wine, then continued along the African coast, taking on water at the Portuguese island outpost of São Tomé. From Africa to the American coast, they encountered difficulties with French corsairs, and part of the fleet was shipwrecked in southern Brazil. Surviving all this, Staden was taken captive by the Tupi. In fact, Staden cleverly used the epidemic to save himself. In 1554 he wrote, "Soon after this I heard weeping and thought the war party had returned, but I found instead that many of

30 Ibid., p. 11.
31 John Hemming, *Red Gold. The Conquest of the Brazilian Indians* (Cambridge, MA: Harvard University Press, 1978), p. 141.
32 Ibid., p. 140.

the savages had fallen sick and their chief, Jeppipo Wasu, told me how the sickness had come and that I had been aware of it." The Tupi chieftain had remembered that earlier Staden told him "that the moon looked angrily on the huts." Staden had indeed, and thought: "Surely it must have been God's Providence that I spoke thus about the moon that night. Then I told him that this had happened because he wanted to eat me, so he promised I should not be harmed if he recovered." The prisoner was gambling with his own life and knew it. Fortunately, Staden won the gamble.

The sequencing of deaths provided in Staden's account is informative; first children succumbed, then the elderly, as is typical in many epidemic bouts. "I went among them laying my hands on their heads, but they began to die; first one of the children, then the chief's old mother, then more of his family. The chief begged me to tell my God to withdraw his wrath. I told him that he would recover his health if he gave up all thoughts of killing me. He ordered all those in his huts to stop mocking me and threatening to eat me. He finally recovered as did one of his wives who had been stricken, but eight of his friends died, as well as others who had treated me with great cruelty." Not long afterward, Staden was asked to cure a Cario slave in the village. The slave had been ill for nine or ten days, and the owner asked Staden to attempt a cure. Staden obliged, first unsuccessfully attempting bloodletting from "the middle vein." Staden told them he would probably die, at which point they decided to kill and eat the slave at once. Staden said, "Do not kill him for he may possibly recover." But they did anyway. "I warned them that as he had been sick they might also become ill if they ate him. Nevertheless one of them cut him up and divided him equally with the others, as is their custom, and they devoured everything except the head and the bowels, which they held in great distaste as he had been sick."[33] It is impossible to calculate total mortality during the epidemic, because there was no accurate population count at the time. Nevertheless, the number of deaths was substantial. Furthermore, one must note that Léry reported an epidemic similar to smallpox that touched only the native Americans but that was much more virulent.[34]

33 Michael Alexander, ed., *Discovering the New World* (New York: Harper & Row, 1976), pp. 115, 117.
34 Warren Dean, "Las poblaciones indígenas del litoral brasileño de São Paulo a Río de Janeiro: Comercio, esclavitud, reducción y extinción," in *Población y mano de obra en América Latina*, ed. Nicolás Sánchez-Albornoz (Madrid: Alianza América, 1985), p. 45.

A little more than a decade later, in 1565, two Jesuit establishments in Espírito Santo were hit by smallpox. Here the number dying was so immense that mass graves had to be dug for the victims. The deaths were so high that the settlements, administered by Jesuits Diogo Iacome and Pero Gonçalves, were virtually abandoned. The two Jesuits remained, giving primary care to those who stayed on. "They were bloodletters, surgeons, doctors and also parish priests and porters" of the dead to the cemeteries. Too many people were sick to help nurse those who had fallen ill or to bury the corpses. Diogo Iacome himself fell victim to the malady after coming down with a fever. "He had been exhausted by such excessive work and consumed with despair at such a sad outcome, watching a populous *aldea* [native settlement] that he loved dearly so rapidly undone, ravaged and abandoned," reported the author of one chronicle.[35] How could such devastation be explained to people recently brought to Christianity and the rite of baptism? The Jesuit Anchieta attempted to expound on what he discerned as God's plan as he inspected the ravaged Espírito Santo hamlets. He "wept with the Indians over their miseries. With his customary eloquence, and in the Brazilian language, he exhorted them to bear that scourge with patience."[36] The Jesuit believed that the pestilence was the will of God, and that the intent was to give eternal salvation to those who were suffering. Dean explains the rational yet ironic position of clergymen who were ministering to the afflicted. The evil were swept away by the disease, suffering the "punishment of God," whereas the already Christianized were "called to Him."[37]

The destruction was viewed differently by some Amerindians who were determined to eradicate the foreigners. The messianic movement of the Santidade was spurred on by the shaman Santo and was a reaction against Portuguese domination with its slavery and "civilization." The Indians rejected the outsiders and called for a return to the old order, in a movement reminiscent of the Taki Onqoy cult of the central Andean highlands during the same decade. Focused in the Bahia district and growing rapidly during the 1562–63 epidemics, the followers believed that "their god would free them from slavery and make them masters of the white people, who would become their slaves." They were admonished not to plant, for food would grow without labor, and "white people would be turned into game for them

35 Hemming, *Red Gold*, p. 145.   36 Ibid., p. 147.
37 Dean, "Poblaciones indígenas del litoral brasileño," p. 46.

to eat." In 1564 Jesuit João Pereira was almost murdered by his Indians as he tried to stop them from fleeing the oncoming epidemic. The movement gathered momentum and continued as a regional force into the next century.[38]

Dean pointed to possible seasonality of the Brazilian epidemics of the 1560s, noting that most outbreaks occurred from March to June, which is fall in this region south of the equator. A variety of factors may have contributed to a higher incidence: the coming of vessels from Europe, lowering temperatures, or a lessening of protein sources. Dean argued that epidemics in the subtropical climate may continue extended throughout the year.[39] Other epidemics swept Brazil during the latter part of the century. Jesuit settlements at Bahia were "being devastated by smallpox and measles" around 1575, with much mortality.[40] Dean attributes part of the spread of epidemics to the almost insatiable demand for Indian slaves. "The cycle of epidemics accelerated as a result of nearly constant raiding. In the late 1570s epidemics again provoked severe labor shortages on the coastal plantations." Slave raids led to Indian uprisings and further deaths.

The importation of Africans for slave labor in the sugar plantations along the coast accelerated sharply in the last quarter of the century. But curiously, the larger numbers, up to 40,000 in the years from 1576 to 1600, did not result in recorded pandemics along the Brazilian coast. Such would not be the case in the seventeenth and eighteenth centuries, when there developed a direct and strong link between the slave trade and smallpox introduction. It has been noted that in 1585 suspected smallpox erupted in the city of Ilhéus. A smallpox epidemic reportedly coincided with conflict between the Portuguese and French and the Indian allies of each in Paraíba in 1597. At its peak, ten to twelve Indians were dying daily from smallpox, forcing the Portuguese commander to suspend military operations. It is possible that the source of this epidemic was a French ship that attacked a Portuguese trading station at Arguin off the Sahara coast. The ship carried on board an active smallpox infection that reached Bahia.[41] Two years later in 1599 a Spanish ship on the way to Buenos Aires stopped at

38 Hemming, *Red Gold*, pp. 143, 157.
39 Dean, "Indigenous Populations," p. 22.   40 Hemming, *Red Gold*, p. 175.
41 Dauril Alden and Joseph C. Miller, "Unwanted Cargoes: The Origin and Dissemination of Smallpox via the Slave Trade, c. 1560–1830," in *The African Exchange. Toward a Biological History of Black People*, ed. Kenneth F. Kiple (Durham: Duke University Press, 1987), pp. 44–45.

Rio de Janeiro. According to the English traveler Anthony Knivet, the crew carried "a disease . . . like the meazels [sic], but as bad as the plague," that led to the demise of "above three thousand Indians and Portugals" in a brief but tragic period of three months.[42]

The demographic consequences of the biological exchange were catastrophic along Brazil's coast, as in other lowland yet reasonably densely populated districts of tropical and subtropical America. By the end of the sixteenth century, according to Dean, "the Tupinamba were nearly extinct on the littoral of Rio de Janeiro, and the Tupiniquim were nearly extinct on the São Paulo littoral."[43] Disease here, as elsewhere, was just one of several factors that led to the demise of Amerindian peoples. Warfare and slaving expeditions were other factors, as was the escape of coastal residents into the vast interior. Because various Europeans were involved in reconnaissance and early exploitation of the coast's resources, especially brazilwood for textile dyes, and because the Portuguese were more lax in their administration and control over local peoples, our knowledge of the Brazilian case is not as complete as for other countries.

Southern North America

The vastness of the Amazonian subcontinent of South America is mirrored by another subcontinent in the northern hemisphere, the Mississippian. The two are entirely different ecologically; only the fact that they are parts of two of the earth's greatest river basins unites them. Both regions were reconnoitered early, although imperfectly, by European explorers who were making their discoveries from the fringes. The Spanish in the south followed up Juan Ponce de León's superficial exploration of Florida's coasts with subsequent efforts, including the Hernando de Soto expedition of 1538–42. Members of the second group reached the Mississippi River and realized the vastness of the continent's interior. In several months of wanderings that took them from the coast near what is today Tampa to as far north as present Chattanooga, then across the Mississippi, the Spanish and a group of Indian allies encountered groups that had already suffered the ravages of European disease.

---

42 Samuel Purchas, Hakluytus Postumus, or Purchas His Pilgrimes, 20 vols. (Glasgow: Maclehose, 1906), 16:237.
43 Dean, "Indigenous Populations," p. 23.

The expedition of Alvar Núñez Cabeza de Vaca and his party allowed for transfer of disease between Spaniards and Amerindians. He frequently mentioned illnesses in his account, especially those that afflicted the often starving Europeans. Although the evidence he provides is inconclusive, it is suggestive of health conditions in general. The odyssey began near Tampa Bay on 14 April 1528, with a group of 300 under the leadership of Governor Pánfilo de Narváez. Of that number only four would live to return to "civilization" several years later. Weakened by hunger, illness, and Indian attacks, the Spanish decided when they entered the territory of the Apalachee in northern Florida to return to the Gulf Coast and to construct small vessels in an attempt to continue to New Spain, sailing along the coast. Cabeza de Vaca reported at this juncture that there were "many others sick," and shortly later, "there were not enough horses to carry the men who were sick, nor did we know what cure to apply, for they grew worse every day."[44] He lamented that "a third of our people were very ill, and since sickness was increasing by the hour, we were sure that all of us were going to succumb to it." Before they began to sail along the coast, "more than forty men had died of illness and hunger."[45] They were shipwrecked on the coast of Texas near present-day Galveston in November 1528, and began their journey along the coast and overland intending to head in the general direction of Mexico. By then, only a handful of Spaniards remained: "Within a very short time only fifteen of the eighty men from both parties who had reached the island were left alive; and after the death of these men, a stomach ailment afflicted the Indians of the land from which half of them died."[46] As happened elsewhere, the outsiders were associated in the popular mind with disease and death. "They believed that it was we

44 Enrique Pupo-Walker, ed., *Castaways. The Narrative of Alvar Núñez Cabeza de Vaca* (Berkeley: University of California Press, 1993), pp. 26–27.
45 Ibid., pp. 28, 30; Henry F. Dobyns, *Their Number Become Thinned: Native American Population Dynamics in Eastern North America* (Knoxville: University of Tennessee Press, 1983), p. 262, argues that it was typhoid fever: "Cabeza de Vaca emphasized a disordered stomach as a symptom, making typhoid a likely diagnosis." Covey says it was malaria; see William T. Pilkington, ed., *Epilogue: Cabeza de Vaca's Adventures in the Unknown Interior of North America*, trans. Cyclone Covey (Albuquerque: University of New Mexico Press, 1984), p. 44. It could have been something entirely different.
46 Pupo-Walker, *Castaways*, p. 46; Pilkington, *Epilogue: Cabeza de Vaca's Adventures*, p. 60; Covey opines that the Spaniards passed on dysentery to the natives.

who were killing them," chronicled Cabeza de Vaca, "and they were wholly convinced of this, they agreed among themselves to kill those of us who were left."[47] On the basis of this evidence, Lawrence E. Aten concluded that "almost from the moment of Cabeza de Vaca's arrival on the Texas coast in 1528, natives began dying from disease introduced by Europeans."[48] There is suggestion of a disease element, but unfortunately the evidence fails to support conclusive identification. Cabeza de Vaca frequently complained about mosquito infestations along the Gulf Coast and into the interior. "In that land we encountered a very large number of mosquitoes of three different kinds, which are very bad and annoying, and during all the rest of the summer they gave us great trouble. . . . And when they [the Indians] leave, they are so bitten by mosquitoes that you would think they had the disease of Saint Lazarus the Leper."[49] At a point in the journey, Cabeza de Vaca and his companions became medicine men, doctors, and survived in part by successfully curing ill Amerindians. At one place he reported that they "took me to heal many others who were lying in a stupor."[50] As their fame as healers spread, they were asked to cure one group after another. "And there they joined other Indians who are called Arbadaos; and we found these very ill and skinny and swollen-bellied, so much so that we were astonished."[51] A number of diseases could have been involved: encephalitis, malaria, even typhoid. Finally nearing the end of the long journey, in 1536, the survivors began to approach the long frontier of New Spain. Still to the north of the settlement line, Cabeza de Vaca noted that they traveled extensively but found the country empty "because those who dwelt in it were fleeing to the mountains, not daring to have houses or cultivate the land for fear of the Christians. It made us extremely sad to see how fertile the land was, and very beautiful, and

47 Pupo-Walker, Castaways, p. 46.
48 Lawrence E. Aten, Indians of the Upper Texas Coast (New York: Academic Press, 1983), pp. 55, 59.
49 Pupo-Walker, Castaways, pp. 62–63.
50 Ibid., p. 72. Another translator renders it as "sick of a stupor" [Buckingham Smith, Relation of Alvar Núñez Cabeça de Vaca (New York: J. Munsell, 1871), p. 122]. Meningitis and encephalitis are possible candidates for the sickness described in the account.
51 Pupo-Walker, Castaways, p. 75. Kiple (1996, personal communication) suggests the possibility of malaria. The distended stomachs could result from swollen spleens. Typhoid also can lead to a swollen spleen and liver.

very full of springs and rivers, and to see every place deserted and burned villages, and the people so thin and ill, all of them fled and hidden."[52]

Later, in 1541 a large party of up to 1,500 under Francisco Vázquez de Coronado, searching for large cities and precious metals, explored the Rio Grande, then marched onward into the Plains, reaching what is now Kansas. Almost simultaneously, the Hernando de Soto forces and Moscoso passed through what is now east Texas and Oklahoma. None were able to find anything of immediate value in that vast region. The Spanish discoveries of substantial silver deposits at Zacatecas in northern central Mexico in 1545 and elsewhere led to virtual abandonment of the less promising regions, such as the far northern borderlands of New Spain. Further penetration of the Plains and desert country came much later and was associated with missionary efforts, defense from Indian attacks, or protection of the fringes of the Spanish empire in America from encroachments by other European powers. The Oñate expedition resulted in the founding of Santa Fé in 1598. From then on there is archaeological evidence of Spanish trade goods arriving on the Plains.

The rough outlines of Florida, initially thought to be an island, were known by the Europeans by 1500, for by then some features regularly begin to appear on maps. Mapping implies sailing along the coast, with probable stops to search for fresh water and safe harbors. Furthermore, the southeast coast of Florida was dangerous for sailing, and many ships went to the bottom, blown off course during storms or accidentally hitting the sharp coral reefs of the keys. This dangerous island area was labeled on the Spanish charts as the "martyrs," indicating the dangers of coming in too close to the shore. The introduction of Old World disease organisms might have taken place early, following shipwrecks, but we cannot definitely say this was the case. Contact could even have taken place via native trade routes. The arguments of historians, anthropologists, and archaeologists are quite heated on this point. Dobyns persists in the belief that contact occurred between the peoples of Florida and Cuba. He argues that "they became especially vulnerable after Spaniards colonized Cuba, because its people and the South Florida Calusa seem to have kept up regular communication." Furthermore, according to Dobyns, the Calusa "traded with Bahama

52 Pupo-Walker, *Castaways*, p. 107.

Islanders."[53] Although the case is hotly contested, there is little doubt that as the native population of Hispaniola declined, the Spanish sailed in search of Indian laborers to replace them. Nearby islands were quickly denuded of people; the mainlands came next. Some slaving expeditions probably did reach Florida's southern coasts prior to the enactment of the Laws of Burgos of 1512, which were intended to protect the Amerindian from the worst abuses of the colonial regime.

In 1513, Juan Ponce de León made the first serious Spanish attempt at Florida exploration; his ostensible purpose was location of a fabled "fountain of youth," but it was likely that slaves or precious metals were the real reasons for the expedition. The expedition landed on Florida's upper east coast in early April, then coasted southward to the keys, and continued up the west coast to perhaps present-day Pensacola. On their return trip toward Cuba, there was a deadly military encounter between Europeans and the Amerindians near Charlotte Bay in late May 1513. Another recorded contact took place in 1517, when the fleet of Francisco Hernández de Córdova was blown by storm onto Florida's west coast on the return from the Yucatán to Cuba. Alonso Alvarez de Pineda discovered in an exploratory mission that reached Mobile Bay in 1519 that Florida was not an island but was attached to the mainland. This was, as we have seen, a period when the Greater Antilles were being decimated by the first smallpox pandemic. A second trip was made by Ponce de León in 1521; it ended in failure, for the leader was wounded near Charlotte Harbor and died following his return to Havana. This second Ponce de León voyage came near the end of the famous first smallpox pandemic.[54] Dobyns posits that the epidemic entered Florida, if not by direct Spanish contact, then by transfer from the islands by Calusa traders or through the Gulf coastal route, which was, in the words of Dobyns, "a continental-margin canoe trade route."[55] According to Smith, the 1521 expedition was characterized by illness: "Significantly, many of the colonists fell ill from an unidentified disease, which the Indians possibly also contracted."[56]

53 Dobyns, Their Number, pp. 250, 259.
54 Michael V. Gannon, The Cross in the Sand: The Early Catholic Church in Florida, 1513–1870 (Gainesville: University of Florida Press, 1965), pp. 1–3.
55 Dobyns, Their Number, p. 260.
56 Marvin T. Smith, Archaeology of Aboriginal Culture Change in the Interior Southeast, Depopulation during the Early Historic Period (Gainesville: University of Florida Press, 1991), p. 55.

A major settlement attempt was made in 1521 on the east Florida coast under orders of Lucas Vázquez de Ayllón, a royal official at Santo Domingo. Ayllón commissioned the effort under Francisco Gordillo and Pedro de Quejo, who gave promising reports on a supposedly rich land named Chicora and located somewhere in the Carolinas district. Much more important was the 1526 settlement attempt directly under Ayllón that involved 600 men, women, and African slaves. The colony, named San Miguel de Gualdape, lasted three brief months, just enough time to construct small houses and a chapel. With the cold of approaching winter, lack of food, and sickness, the settlement failed. By the time the decision was made to abandon the colony and return to Santo Domingo, only 150 of the original 600 settlers remained. The slaves may have been left behind.[57]

Another avenue of infection might have stemmed from the 1528 expedition of Pánfilo de Narváez in a small contingent that sailed back to Cuba for supplies, then returned to Charlotte Harbor. Four men were left ashore and were executed by the Calusa within three days, but eighteen-year-old Juan Ortíz was spared, lived on as a slave, then escaped to survive under the protection of nearby Chief Mocoso. He was liberated by Hernando de Soto in 1539, and according to Dobyns might have been the one to carry disease from Cuba to south Florida in 1528.[58]

The Hernando de Soto expedition was large enough and lasted long enough to cause great ecological damage, although disease had earlier taken its toll. Reaching Cofitachique north of the Savannah River in 1540, the Soto expedition found evidence that surrounding communities had been pummelled recently by disease. The account by the Gentleman of Elvas confirms this possibility: "About this place, from half a league to a league off, were large vacant towns grown up in grass that appeared as if no people had lived in them for a long time. The Indians said that, two years before, there had been a pest in the land, and that the inhabitants had moved away to other towns."[59]

---

57 Paul E. Hoffman, *New Andalucia and a Way to the Orient: The American Southeast during the Sixteenth Century* (Baton Rouge: Louisiana State University Press, 1990), pp. 3–15, 60–80.

58 Dobyns, *Their Number*, p. 262; Gannon, *Cross in the Sand*, pp. 7–9; Suzanne and Paul Fish, "Historic Demography and Ethnographic Analogy," *Early Georgia* 7(1979):29–43.

59 Ann F. Ramenofsky, *Vectors of Death: The Archaeology of European Contact* (Albuquerque: University of New Mexico Press, 1987), p. 67.

The account of the conquest of Florida compiled by Garcilaso de la Vega, relates that "they had little food because a great pestilence with many consequent deaths had ravaged their province during the past year, a pestilence from which their town alone had been free. For this reason the inhabitants of the other villages of that province had fled to the forests without sowing their fields. And now, although the disease had passed, these people had not yet been gathered to their homes and towns."[60]

Other attempts to settle Florida could have led to the introduction of foreign pathogens. In 1547 Dominican Luis Cáncer de Barbastro, while a missionary in Guatemala, decided to bring Christianity to Florida. It was not until May 1549 that he was able to reach the coast, near Tampa Bay, where he and several others suffered martyrdom. The Cáncer group came across another Spaniard, Juan Muñoz, who had lived among the natives of Florida for a decade, probably having been captured from the Soto forces. Muñoz escaped captivity to join the Spaniards and provided vital testimony on local conditions. Given the fierce opposition of the Indians and learning that there was no precious metal to be found in the vicinity, the forces returned to Mexico. The next decade a new major expedition under Tristán de Luna y Arellano, composed of about 1,500 men, women, and children, left Veracruz for Florida, landing at Pensacola Bay in August 1559. The fleet was devastated by a hurricane, and most supplies were destroyed. Part of the group went inland to the village of Nanipacana, another to a place called Coosa. Some had been with Soto two decades earlier, and the place seemed different, with a smaller population and less food. The weakened survivors stayed on for a year and a half, before they also gave up and returned to Mexico. Thus, before the foundation of St. Augustine on Florida's east coast in 1565, there had been several major Spanish efforts at intervals of roughly a decade that left a mark on the human landscape of Florida. Marvin T. Smith suggests that the region around Coosa "had no doubt lost population to European disease, but apparently the population had stabilized in the period between the visits of Soto and Luna."[61]

The northern sector of Spanish Florida came under one more important reconnaissance before the end of the century. Captain Juan

60 John Grier Varner and Jeannette Johnson Varner, trans. and ed., *The Florida of the Inca by Garcilaso de la Vega* (Austin: University of Texas Press, 1988), p. 298.

61 Smith, *Archaeology of Aboriginal Culture Change*, pp. 11–12; Hoffman, *New Andalucia*, pp. 99–101, 153–59, 169–72.

Pardo conducted two investigations of the interior of Santa Elena between 1566 and 1568. He took a route parallel to that of Soto three decades before, and scribe Juan de la Bandera kept a record of the route. The extent of the changes that had transpired in a brief thirty years was amazing. When Soto saw the region, it was, according to archaeologist Marvin T. Smith, an era of "flourishing complex chiefdoms, large towns, dense populations, high levels of military organization, complex religion, and elites marked by sumptuary rules." Smith later concluded that the area described by sixteenth-century Spanish explorers was very distinct from what existed in "the late seventeenth and eighteenth centuries. By that time, the large populations had been reduced by disease and the chiefdoms had been reduced to less complex units."[62]

We have already noted the occurrence of several bouts of disease along the east coast of Florida. In St. Augustine there was an unidentified epidemic in the summer of 1596, for the following year the new governor, Gonzalo Méndez de Canzo, described how well the recently organized hospital had helped to prevent the death of many soldiers, Indians, and Blacks.[63] In 1596 a new expedition set out into the backlands from the Franciscan missionary base at Guale (St. Catherine's Island). Again, there was indication of a less dense population than earlier. The first seven days the group under Gaspar de Salas passed through "deserted" territory that earlier had been populated.[64]

In the southwest of what is today the United States and northwestern Mexico, disease also seems to have swept far ahead of conquest. Reff has developed a disease chronology for the region, noting sixteen widespread disease outbreaks from 1530 to 1653. Failing to find direct evidence of the spread of the first smallpox pandemic into the region, he nonetheless reports malaria, dysentery, and perhaps typhoid in 1530–31, measles from 1530 to 1534, perhaps typhus in the period 1545–48. Dobyns, Stoffle, and Jones report bubonic plague in 1545, and typhus, typhoid, and dysentery from 1576 to 1581.[65] Dobyns, Stoffle, and Jones suggested the possible passage of an epidemic of smallpox among the Pueblo in 1564. With the arrival of the Jesuits in the region in 1591, record keeping allows for a more concrete and accurate epidemic series to be generated by modern historians. By

62 Ibid., pp. 12–13.   63 Dobyns, *Their Number*, p. 278.

64 Smith, *Archaeology of Aboriginal Culture Change*, p. 15.

65 Daniel T. Reff, *Disease, Depopulation, and Culture Change in Northwestern New Spain, 1518–1764* (Salt Lake City: University of Utah Press, 1991), pp. 103–77.

then, according to Reff, the Black Robes found "only vestiges of once populous and developed cultures. . . . Most native populations were reduced by 30 to over 50 percent prior to sustained contact with the Jesuits."[66] Their policy of settlement, or *congregaciones*, had the same devastating consequences as concentration into the *aldeas* in Brazil or into the *reducciones* of Viceroy Toledo in Peru: Higher population densities concurrently enhanced epidemic mortality. The expansion of Spanish mining into Durango and southern Chihuahua from 1546, with a much higher concentration of Europeans, created the focal points for the penetration of infectious disease. Here, as in Brazil, natives came to believe that the clergymen were the true cause of death. Various ailments coincided chronologically with the foundation of the Jesuit missions in 1591; there were measles among the Pueblo in 1592 and smallpox and measles in the region in 1593. In 1594 there was smallpox. As Lovell commented, "A backlash was inevitable." The wrath of the natives turned on the Jesuits. During a pastoral inspection of Tovoropa, the Indians rose on 11 July 1594. They blamed the many deaths of their people on the coming of the Black Robes, burned the church, and killed Friar Gonzalo de Tapia. "After setting the church on fire, they stuck Father Gonzalo's head on a pole and paraded it on a circuit of neighboring settlements."[67]

The St. Lawrence and Upper Mississippi Valleys

The vast interior of northeastern North America, including the Upper Mississippi, came under relatively early contact and penetration from Newfoundland and the St. Lawrence and Hudson River valleys. Between 1497 and 1534 there were at least five French or Portuguese expeditions to the Gulf of St. Lawrence area that initiated sporadic contact with the people along the shore. John Cabot, sailing for the English, had landed on Newfoundland in June 1497 and probably coasted farther to the south. Two voyages of the Portuguese, under Gaspar Corte-Real and his brother Miguel in 1500 and 1501, coasted mainland Canada. Fifty-seven natives were captured in Newfoundland on the second expedition and taken to Europe. Sebastian Cabot, John

66 Ibid., pp. 15–16.
67 George W. Lovell, " 'Heavy Shadows and Black Night': Disease and Depopulation in Colonial Spanish America," in *Annals of the Association of American Geographers* 82(1992):433.

Cabot's son, sailed for England in 1508 or 1509 and may have touched Hudson Bay. Key to northern movement into the interior were the expeditions of Jacques Cartier, whose 1534 voyage up the St. Lawrence was followed by others. In New France about fifty Stadaconan Indians died during an epidemic in December 1535. About the same time, twenty-five Europeans died from an unidentified sickness.[68] According to one account, Chief Hochelaga believed the foreigners might be able to effect a cure. Cartier, sensing possible advantage, recited Christian texts in French and played the role of a shaman so persuasively that "at once many sick persons, some blind, others with but one eye, others lame or impotent and others again so extremely old that their eyelids hung down to their cheeks, were brought in and set down or laid out near the Captain, in order that he might lay lands upon them, so that one would have thought Christ had come down to earth to heal them." As Axtell points out, the natives of the St. Lawrence quickly associated the outsiders with the power of sickness and healing, comparable to that of the indigenous shamans. Both "were thought to wield powers of life and death."[69]

By 1541, after three expeditions to the area, two small temporary forts had been constructed by the French. Furthermore, for disease transfer it is significant that after 1497 there was regular contact between Amerindians and the fishing fleets off the Grand Banks, with voyages in most years by English, French, and Portuguese fishermen. Some barter between Old and New World peoples took place during the summer months, particularly after dry fishing, which required drying the lightly salted codfish in the open, became prevalent. Also, between 1540 and 1610 Portuguese whaling settlements dotted the Labrador coast, and although these too were seasonal affairs, some exchanges with nearby native Americans occurred.

The disease experience of the natives surrounding the Roanoke settlement of the English has already been examined, because it seems part of a broader pandemic related to the Drake expedition when it returned from the Caribbean. Another colony was attempted at Sable

68 Russell Thornton, *American Indian Holocaust and Survival: A Population History since 1492* (Norman: University of Oklahoma Press, 1987), p. 14; Ramenofsky, *Vectors of Death*, p. 98.
69 James Axtell, *The Invasion from Within. The Contest of Cultures in Colonial North America* (New York: Oxford University Press, 1985), p. 10. The quotation on Cartier and Chief Hochelaga comes from H. P. Biggar, ed., *The Voyages of Jacques Cartier* (Ottawa: F. A. Acland, 1924), pp. 56, 62, 162–63.

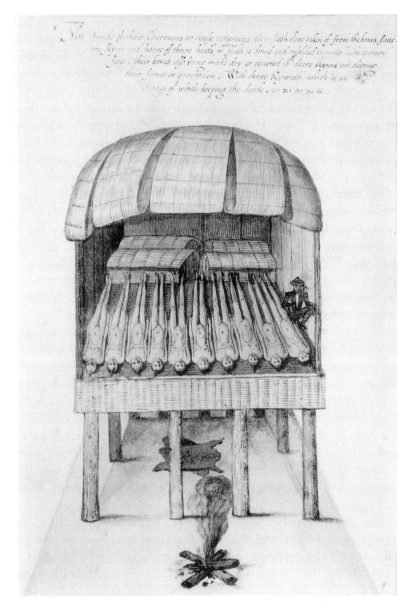

Figure 4.1. Indian charnel house at Secoton, 1585, from Paul Hulton, *America 1585: The Complete Drawings of John White*, pl. 38.

Island, Nova Scotia, two years before the century's end. By the end of the sixteenth century, the basic outlines of settlement had been laid that were to distinguish both the French and English experience in North America from that of the Spanish and the Portuguese. It is clear that before 1600 European penetration of northeastern North America took place, but no permanent year-round settlements had been established. Nonetheless, the regular summer posts and the trade in furs and European commodities – knives, fishhooks, mirrors, bells, metal arrow points – permitted continuous exchange of not only goods but also infections. Only the lack of interest in careful record keeping meant that the major episodes of disease were not documented. Near the beginning of the seventeenth century both the French and English, and later the Dutch, would set up permanent colonies along the Atlantic Coast. By that time, the numbers of native Americans living in those regions had already declined to the point that they could put up little resistance to outside pressure. What the French and English saw as virgin land had already, in the previous century, been denuded of people. The remnants were already weakened and were easy prey for foreign settlers. Disease conquest preceded the encroachment of the colonists, and by the time the *Mayflower* touched American shores, that conquest was already largely complete.

CHAPTER FIVE

New Arrivals

PEOPLES AND ILLNESSES
FROM 1600 to 1650

Lord put an end to this quarrel by smiting them with smallpox.
. . . Thus did the Lord allay their quarrelsome spirit and make
room for the following part of his army.

William Wood, New England, 1634

The filthy smell and stench which came from them which lay
sick of this disease was enough to infect the rest of the house,
and all that came to see them. . . . Very few Spaniards were
infected by this contagion; but the Indians were generally taken
with it.

Thomas Gage, Guatemala

Terror was universal. The contagion increased as autumn advanced; and when winter came, its ravages were appalling. The
season of the Huron festivity was turned to a season of mourning;
and such was the despondency and dismay, that suicides became
frequent.

French Canada, 1636

By the beginning of the seventeenth century, some arthropod-
transmitted illnesses such as typhus, the plague, and perhaps malaria,
introduced from the Old World to the New, had settled down to an
endemic existence. The same may have been true of some of the
acutely infectious communicable diseases. Epidemics flared up from
time to time at various places, sometimes breaking out when local
conditions of health and nutrition deteriorated. Crop failures resulting
from drought, insect infestations, or blight at times caused enough

starvation to weaken the population to the point at which disease could prosper. A localized epidemic explosion would result, often with high mortality. In some places, such as the central plateau of Mexico, crop productivity was often not great, and famine was always a threat. The balance between food resources and population in Mexico was frequently broken, with catastrophic economic and social consequences. Central Mexico's population recovery was at first a halting affair, with growth alternating with short but profound reverses. In regions of the Americas with less likelihood of food failure, the halt in the collapse of native populations and demographic recovery frequently began earlier.

SMALLPOX IN THE SECOND DECADE OF THE SEVENTEENTH CENTURY

Some American epidemics during the initial half of the seventeenth century were widespread enough to be rightly identified as pandemics. The compound smallpox and measles epidemic of the mid-1610s was probably one of these widely dispersed series. For example, Prem found evidence of the appearance of disease in the central valley of Mexico in 1613, but more important, there were smallpox and measles from 1615 to 1616.[1] Reff recorded significant smallpox and perhaps measles outbreaks in northwestern Mexico in 1616 that continued into 1617. Indeed, using Jesuit materials, Reff noted various maladies: measles, smallpox, pneumonia, and typhus, among others, finding evidence in mission records for peak years of mortality in 1601–2, 1607–8, 1612–13, 1617, and 1623–25.[2]

Lovell noted illnesses in Guatemala during this period but was unable to identify specific diseases. Testimony from around 1613 indicated sick Indians in Todos Santos Cuchumatán, with a *peste general* in Santiago de Guatemala in 1614. Then, sick Indians were reported in San Martín Cuchumatán in 1617. In the following year, in several towns in Chiapas, there was a decrease in the population due to

1 Hanns J. Prem, "Disease Outbreaks in Central Mexico during the Sixteenth Century," in *The Secret Judgments of God: Native Peoples and Old World Disease in Colonial Spanish America*, ed. Noble David Cook and W. George Lovell (Norman: University of Oklahoma Press, 1992), p. 43.
2 Daniel T. Reff, "Culture Shock in Northwestern New Spain, 1518–1764," in *Disease and Demography in the Americas*, ed. John W. Verano and Douglas H. Ubelaker (Washington, DC: Smithsonian Institution Press, 1992), p. 268.

Table 5.1. *Major Guatemalan epidemics,*
1600–1650

1607–8	Typhus (*enfermedad general*)
1620s	Smallpox (*peste general*)
1631–32	Typhus
1650	"Plague"

Source: Lovell, "Disease in Early Colonial
Guatemala," p. 59.

"sicknesses and deaths of the natives."[3] Newson points out that farther
to the south in Nicaragua in 1617 "smallpox, typhus, and measles were
reported as having killed many Indians."[4] (See Table 5.1.)

In Andean America the series of epidemic episodes in the second
decade of the new century were equally complex. There were several
points of entry for foreign pathogens; the port of Cartagena, with its
important slave market, was especially vulnerable. According to the
Annual Report of the Jesuits for 1611, a ship with infected slaves that
arrived from the Cape Verde Islands was prevented from unloading.
According to the report, many slaves were suffering from "smallpox,
measles, and *tabardillo* (typhus)." In spite of quarantine, the Jesuit
Alonso de Sandoval went aboard to administer the rites of the church
and must have contributed to the spread of contagion.[5]

In the Audiencia of Quito measles appeared in 1611, along with
typhus, according to one report. These diseases continued into 1612,
when scarlet fever also broke out. In 1618 a severe strain of measles
hit children especially hard.[6] Measles swept central Colombia in
1617–18. Mortality approached one out of five for the native American population, although as elsewhere, the impact of measles on

---

3 W. George Lovell, "Disease and Depopulation in Early Colonial Guatemala," in
   Secret Judgments, ed. Cook and Lovell, p. 64.
4 Linda A. Newson, *Indian Survival in Colonial Nicaragua* (Norman: University of
   Oklahoma Press, 1987), p. 248.
5 Alonso de Sandoval, *De Instaurando Aethiopium Salute . . .* (Bogotá: Empresa
   Nacional de Publicaciones, 1956), pp. 569–70; Antonio Astrain, *Historia de la
   compañía de Jesús en la asistencia de España* (Madrid: Administración de Razón y
   Fé, 1913), 4:600.
6 Linda A. Newson, *Life and Death in Early Colonial Ecuador* (Norman: University
   of Oklahoma Press, 1995), p. 151.

peninsular-born Spaniards was minimal.[7] Chandler noted that the measles epidemic of 1616 resulted in such massive mortality that the mines of Los Remedios and Zaragoza in Colombia were virtually abandoned.[8]

Measles seems to have been generalized in the viceroyalty of Peru in 1618, for the king wrote to Viceroy Esquilache to congratulate him on the success he had in limiting the epidemic's impact there. The following year, 1619, saw measles with high mortality in Copacabana on Lake Titicaca.[9] This was most likely a continuation of the epidemic into the southern Andean region. It seems that 1619 saw *alfombrilla* (likely identification is rubella) in both northern and southern Peru.[10] Covarrubias defines it the same as *alhombra*. According to him, it is characterized by "some blotches that tend to appear on the face, which are called *alhombra*, because they are caused by an abundance of blood and heat, making that part [of the body] very colored." Father Calancha mentions that the epidemic had depopulated Trujillo, and Ramos Gavilán reports that it had a significant impact on the south in the region around Potosí. The same year crickets were plentiful and "some reddish mice" covered the fields; the appearance of insects and rodents suggests the possibility of bubonic plague.[11] Potosí was especially afflicted by disease between May and August of 1619. The corregidor reported that temporary hospitals had been established in nearby Indian settlements, which had helped to reduce mortality. Bakewell notes that "worms that consumed the intestines 'and other parts' were an especially nasty accompaniment to this sickness, though they were successfully combatted with clysters."[12] Farther south, smallpox was reported in the spring of 1619 in Chile, where approximately 50,000

---

7 Juan A. Villamarin and Judith E. Villamarin, "Epidemic Disease in the Sabana de Bogotá, 1536–1810," in *Secret Judgments*, ed. Cook and Lovell, pp. 122–23.

8 David L. Chandler, *Health and Slavery in Colonial Colombia* (New York: Arno Press, 1981), p. 128.

9 Archivo General de Indias, Seville, Lima 571/72, Madrid, 28 March 1620; Juan B. Lastres, *Historia de la medicina peruana*, 3 vols. (Lima: San Marcos, 1951), 2:179.

10 Henry F. Dobyns, "An Outline of Andean Epidemic History to 1720," *Bulletin of the History of Medicine* 37 (1963):509.

11 Lastres, *Historia de la medicina peruana*, 2:180.

12 Peter Bakewell, *Miners of the Red Mountain. Indian Labor in Potosí, 1545–1650* (Albuquerque: University of New Mexico Press, 1984), p. 110; Archivo General de Indias, Seville, Lima 38 and Charcas 52.

Table 5.2. *Principal epidemic appearances in America,*
1600–1650

Mesoamerica		Andean America	
1604	Measles, typhus, mumps	1606	Diphtheria
1613–17	Smallpox, measles,	1611–14	Measles, typhus, diphtheria
	typhus	1618	Measles
1631–32	Typhus	1630–33	Typhus
1647–49	Yellow fever, Caribbean	1651	Smallpox

people reportedly died. In the autumn of 1620 smallpox was again noted in Chile.[13] (See Table 5.2.)

Along the eastern coast of Brazil in 1613, smallpox infected slaves in Rio de Janeiro working on the sugar plantations. At the time most people believed that the source of infection were Africans. This bout may have sputtered out, but in 1616 smallpox and measles lashed the Brazilian northeastern coast. Recent investigation pinpoints the source of original contagion as being "slaves from the Kongo in central Africa and from Allada on the Lower Guinea Coast."[14] The Tupinamba were overwhelmed by smallpox in 1621 at São Luis de Maranhao. It struck with "such virulence that any who caught it – most of whom were Indians – did not survive for more than three days." As it spread, the epidemic wiped out twenty-seven of the most populated Tupinamba towns on the island of Maranhao.[15]

On the Atlantic Coast of North America, a major epidemic was reported for 1612–13. In the region that later became New England, seventeenth-century epidemics are chronicled regularly. The Pawtuckett were hard pressed. Gookin, who wrote about six decades following the historical event, reported that "a very great number of them, were swept away by an epidemical and unwanted sickness, A. 1612–13, about seven or eight years before the English arrived in those parts to

---

13 Dobyns, "Andean Epidemic History," p. 509.
14 Dauril Alden and Joseph C. Miller, "Out of Africa. The Slave Trade and the Transmission of Smallpox to Brazil, 1560–1831," *Journal of Interdisciplinary History* 18(1987):200.
15 John Hemming, *Red Gold: The Conquest of the Brazilian Indians* (Cambridge, MA: Harvard University Press, 1978), pp. 215–16.

settle the colony of New Plymouth."[16] Although no origin is indicated, Ramenofsky suggests that it is probable that the recorded Massachusetts outbreak of 1612–13 derived from Dutch trading vessels going
up the Hudson Valley. Cook argued that the 1612–13 epidemic may
have been the plague, but the record is scant at best.[17] On the other
hand, the epidemic may have been associated with French fur traders
who in 1612 clashed with natives in the Massachusetts Bay area. One
Frenchman was captured and survived, and later reported on his
misadventures. Learning the language, he told his captors that they
would soon suffer, for "God would be angry with them for it, and that
he would in his displeasure destroy them." The Sachem refused to
believe the Frenchman's prediction, but the plague swept the area
shortly afterward. Vaughan suggests that the prophecy "created a new
fear and respect for the power of the white man."[18]

Better information is available for the epidemic outbreak that began
in 1616. According to Cotton Mather, disease swept through New
England, clearing the land "of those pernicious creatures, to make
room for better growth."[19] The European newcomers seemed immune
to the ravages of the contagion, but the native Americans suffered
dearly. In settlements in Maine in the winter of 1616–17, Europeans
slept in the same cabins with dying Indians, but "not one of them ever
felt their heads to ache, while they stayed there."[20] Other Europeans
living in the Boston Bay area wrote later (1622) referring to Indian
mortality during the illness of 1616–17 that they "died in heapes, as
they lay in their houses." Flight seemed to many to be the only road
to salvation: "The living, that were able to shift for themselves, would
runne away and let them dy, and let there Carkases ly above the
ground without burial." Thomas Morton, who described the event,
was shocked by the Bosch-like scene of horror that he witnessed: "And
the bones and skulls upon the several places of their habitations made

---

16 Ann F. Ramenofsky, *Vectors of Death: The Archaeology of European Contact*
   (Albuquerque: University of New Mexico Press, 1987), p. 99.
17 Sherburne F. Cook, "Significance of Disease in the Extinction of the New
   England Indian," *Human Biology* 45(1973):485–508.
18 Alden T. Vaughan, *New England Frontier. Puritans and Indians 1620–1675*
   (Boston: Little, Brown, 1965), p. 60.
19 Alfred W. Crosby, *The Columbian Exchange: Biological and Cultural Consequences of 1492* (Westport, CT: Greenwood Press, 1972), p. 42.
20 Ibid.

such a spectacle after my coming into those partes, that, as I travailed in that Forrest nere the Massachusetts, it seemed to me a new found Golgotha."[21] This description of devastation is reminiscent of the vivid accounts of the plight of those suffering during the first smallpox pandemic when it hit Mexico roughly a century before.

Many of the English settlers did not find the demise of the native Americans to be wholly unwelcome. In 1620, for example, Miles Standish, leader of the Plymouth colony, found only "a few straggling inhabitants, burial places, empty wigwams, and some skeletons."[22] One settler confessed with more pride than guilt that "Thus farre hath the good hand of God favored our beginnings. . . . In sweeping away great multitudes of the natives . . ., a little more before we went thither, that he might make room for us there."[23] Modern specialist Vaughan concurs on the extent of the devastation, for the epidemic was the "most deadly in recorded history to visit that section of the continent. Its path was strewn with the wreckage of tribes that had once been masters of their territories; it left them weak, unprotected and frightened."[24]

What was this illness, or series of sicknesses of 1616–20 that so severely converged on Amerindians of northeastern North America? Some have offered arguments to identify smallpox, others measles, bubonic plague, and even, incorrectly, yellow fever. Regardless of the exact element, the epidemic clearly extracted a large toll in human lives. Given the extremely deadly nature of the series, it would seem that the principal culprit was smallpox in various forms and with generally high levels of mortality. It may have coincided with measles, with age-specific mortality elevated to about 20 percent. If the series had included bubonic plague or typhus, the English would also have

---

21 Thomas Morton, *New England Canaan* (Boston: Prince Society Publications XIV, 1883), pp. 132–33; Vaughan, *New England Frontier*, p. 354, says that a third or more of the native population between the Penobscot River and Narragansett Bay perished. He concluded that there was "violent depopulation" and that in consequence the coast was opened for settlement by others. Furthermore, the epidemic "upset the intertribal balance of power" and led to a new round of native warfare.

22 Russell Thornton, *American Indian Holocaust and Survival: A Population History since 1492* (Norman: University of Oklahoma Press, 1987), p. 71.

23 Ibid.

24 Ibid., p. 21. Vaughan suggests (p. 22) that it "might have been measles, bubonic plague, or even, perhaps, a combination of diseases that hit various tribes simultaneously."

faced noteworthy deaths and would have mentioned the fact, unless of course most of the first settlers had experienced either or both diseases in Holland or England in the years immediately before sailing to New England.[25]

The possible Old World source for the especially virulent strains of smallpox and perhaps measles that reached the Americas during the first decades of the 1600s, as Alden and Miller have demonstrated, was the slave trade. The outbreaks coincided with severe drought in the edge of Saharan West Africa, as well as in Angola. Both famine and illness were reported on the Cape Verde Islands off the African coast in 1620, and the drought may have started earlier. Rainfall was insufficient for crops in Angola from 1614 to 1619, and local conditions were difficult. The fact that ill captives were packed on board cramped vessels that plied the trade between Africa and the Americas during these critical years resulted in especially high slave mortality.[26]

Smallpox, often combined with an outbreak of measles, devastated parts of the Americas in the last half of the second decade of the seventeenth century. The coincidence of the epidemics is close enough to suggest that this was a true pandemic, rather than a series of isolated epidemic episodes. It is informative to remember that the major smallpox pandemics took place in 1518–25, 1576–91, and 1614–20, at approximate, although not exact, fifty-year intervals. Localized epidemics broke out in intervening years, but the major killers appear to have been separated by full generations.

TYPHUS IN THE EARLY 1630s

Typhus swept some but not all regions of the Americas in the early 1630s. The Guatemalan highlands and the northern and central Andean regions of South America were especially hard pressed. Some of our best descriptions of the event come from those who witnessed the epidemic's disastrous passage through Guatemala in 1631–32. The seventeenth-century Dominican Friar Antonio de Molina wrote that "in 1631 there was in this city of Guatemala a very great sickness that

25 Herbert U. Williams, "Epidemics among Indians, 1616–1620," *Johns Hopkins Hospital Bulletin* 20 (1909):340–49.

26 Dauril Alden and Joseph C. Miller, "Unwanted Cargoes: The Origin and Dissemination of Smallpox via the Slave Trade, c. 1560–1830," in *The African Exchange: Toward a Biological History of Black People*, ed. Kenneth F. Kiple (Durham: Duke University Press, 1987), pp. 46–47.

carried off a large number of people." According to him, it extended
from the city into all provinces of Guatemala and also prevailed in
neighboring towns. Mortality was "terrible" in the capital. On 27
April 1632, the city council requested church authorities to call for a
religious procession that would bring about an end to the contagion.[27]

The Englishman Thomas Gage witnessed the outbreak and provided one of the best descriptions of the epidemic and its manifestations. A devout Catholic, Gage was educated by Jesuits in France and
Spain and then joined the Dominican order. His long account of
travels begins with his voyage to the Caribbean, where he landed at
Veracruz to begin the trek to his mission post in Guatemala. Gage's
trip coincided with one of the most serious and general disease outbreaks of the seventeenth century: "All that country was generally
infected with a kind of contagious sickness, almost as infectious as the
plague, which they call *tabardillo*, and was a fever in the very inward
parts and bowels, which scarce continued to the seventh day but
commonly took them away from the world to a grave on the third or
fifth day. The filthy smell and stench which came from them which
lay sick of this disease was enough to infect the rest of the house, and
all that came to see them. It rotted their mouths and tongues, and
made them as black as coal before they died. Very few Spaniards were
infected by this contagion; but the Indians were generally taken with
it."[28] Gage's description is not far from the actual symptoms of typhus.
Typhus is characterized by a fever, followed by a dark rash. There are
three principal forms of the disease: epidemic, or classical; endemic, or
murine; and *tsutsugamushi*. The epidemic form is the most common in
America and is carried by the body louse, *Pendiculus humanus*. Endemic typhus is carried by the flea and has a reduced rate of mortality.
Tsutsugamushi is transmitted through the mite. The causative agent is
Rickettsia prowazekii, which lives in the cells in the gut of the body
louse. The agent is expelled in the feces; the microorganism is capable
of surviving in the dried feces for up to several days. The agent
normally enters the human body through abrasions in the skin, such
as scratches. Incubation lasts from ten to fourteen days. Headache,
appetite loss, general malaise, and fevers characterize the ailment. At
the end of the first week, body temperature peaks and continues

27 Lovell, "Disease in Early Colonial Guatemala," pp. 79–80.
28 Thomas Gage, *The English American: A New Survey of the West Indies* (London:
    Routledge, 1928), p. 291.

elevated to the twelfth day, when, in survivors, it finally descends to normal at about the fourteenth to sixteenth day. A reddish or dark rash of spots about 2 to 5 millimeters in size breaks out on the fourth to sixth day, with some of them being raised above the surrounding skin. Covering the thorax, the rash may appear to resemble a sleeveless cloak, or *tabardillo*, as the Spanish called the ailment. Average mortality ranges from 5 to 25 percent. Mortality is low in children at about 5 percent; for the elderly it can be higher, in the neighborhood of 50 percent.[29]

Gage noted that the epidemic started in Mexico, then moved southward from town to town into Guatemala, following a similar march of locusts the previous year that had lowered crop yields and had led to hunger.[30] Gage ultimately broke with the Dominican order and fled, reaching England in late 1637. He converted to Anglicanism and in 1648 published a travel account that was used to justify English encroachments in the Caribbean under Oliver Cromwell. Gage was correct in his account of typhus, for there is ample evidence that it afflicted central Mexico from 1629 to 1631. Gibson, for example, found evidence that typhus (*cocoliztli*) could be found in all areas, with substantial numbers of deaths. But this term may also be a label for the plague, as recently argued by Malvido and Viesca. Unfortunately the sickness returned in 1633–34, along with a severe cough that was called *chichimeca*.[31] Again, mortality was high.

In South America in 1630–33 an epidemic of exanthematic typhus passed through the population of Colombia with especially devastating consequences. The bout began in Santa Fé de Bogotá, with about one-third of the Indians nearby dying but with overall mortality in the region of about one-fifth.[32] According to Chandler, typhus first entered New Granada in 1629, carried by infected slaves from the coastal port of Cartagena de Indias. The epidemic progressed with greatest ease in the cooler highlands, in part because in tropical humid districts sparse clothing and frequent bathing controlled the number of body

---

29 Noble David Cook and W. George Lovell, "Unraveling the Web of Disease," in *Secret Judgments*, ed. Cook and Lovell, pp. 225–27.

30 Gage, *English American*, p. 291.

31 Charles Gibson, *The Aztecs Under Spanish Rule. A History of the Indians of the Valley of Mexico, 1519–1810* (Stanford: Stanford University Press, 1964), p. 450; Elsa Malvido and Carlos Viesca, "La epidemia de cocoliztli de 1576," *Historias* (México, DF) 11(1985):27–33.

32 Villamarin and Villamarin, "Epidemics in the Sabana de Bogotá," pp. 123–25.

lice and hence reduced the chances for infection. Typhus-related deaths were reported in Lima in September and December of 1629.[33] By 1630 the epidemic reached the area surrounding the capital of Bogotá, where it came to be called the Plague of Santos Gil after the name of the notary who prepared many of the wills of those who had fallen sick. In Santa Fé de Bogotá, a priest named Hazañero described the symptoms in detail: "At first chills and fevers were common and within two days the disease had overcome the head, completely depriving the persons of their senses. It left the victims in such a state that they became incapable of helping themselves, with a loss of appetite, uneasiness, anxiety, vomiting, the body paralyzed, the head aching, the patient powerless even to turn in bed, the heartbeat feeble, the bones aching, the throat ulcerated and the teeth chattering, the patient delirious and the whole body burning up with fever." Mortality was high and was estimated to be half or more of most affected households. All socioeconomic classes were afflicted, although as is all too common during the passage of the great killer epidemics, the weakest economically suffered most. Soriano estimated that "eighty percent of the Indians of the Bogotá plateau died in the epidemic."[34] On the basis of pre- and postepidemic population figures for select districts, and taking into account possible growth between epidemic years, a drop of 20 to 25 percent is more likely. The health consequences were both severe and long-lasting. Some who fell ill never regained their former senses; "others remained crippled or deformed and many were left deaf."[35] The priest Father Hazañero wrote that "this contagion continued for more than two years, and there was no one to sow or harvest the crops. The weak, emaciated and pale men, were made of the stamp of death; it seemed as if they already felt the nearness of the last day of time."[36]

In Ecuador typhus is mentioned as being in Quito in 1634 and 1639. Diego Rodríguez Docampo wrote a description of the district in 1650 and referred to the salubrious consequences of bringing the image of the Virgin of Quinche to the cathedral of Quito in 1634, for he related that event to the end of the "great sickness of *tabardete* that

---

33 Juan Antonio Suardo, *Diario de Lima (1629–1634)* (Lima: Vásquez, 1935), pp. 23, 34.
34 Chandler, *Health and Slavery*, p. 131; Villamarin and Villamarin, "Epidemics in the Sabana de Bogotá," pp. 124–25.
35 Villamarin and Villamarin, "Epidemics in the Sabana de Bogotá," pp. 124–25; Chandler, *Health and Slavery*, p. 132.
36 Villamarin and Villamarin, "Epidemics in the Sabana de Bogotá," p. 125.

swept the province of Quito." When the religious celebrations associated with the transport of the Virgin to the cathedral were finished, the people saw a ball of fire in the sky and general health was returned to the people, according to the account.[37]

The Lima diarist Suardo noted that news was received in Lima on 23 January 1631 of the death of the archbishop of New Granada, from "*esquilencia* that took his life away within ten hours."[38] Although his death might not have been the consequence of exanthematic typhus, Suardo pointed out a strong indication of the spread of the disease in a letter from the Ciudad de la Plata that reached Lima on 29 July 1630. The messenger had left the Royal Audiencia in La Plata on 29 June, carrying with him news from the governor of Buenos Aires that the Dutch had successfully taken Pernambuco with a fleet of sixty-nine warships. He also reported that "the President of the Audiencia, Licentiate Martín Egues y Beaumonte, was approaching death from a severe case of pestilential *tabardillo* [typhus] that had removed his senses." A subsequent letter reached Lima on 14 August confirming the president's untimely demise.[39]

Typhus may also have entered the upper Uruguay River region, where the Jesuits had been settling, or "reducing," Indians into European-style towns in the early seventeenth century. Concurrent with forced settlement, as in the case of the Andean area under Viceroy Francisco de Toledo half a century earlier, came disease and death. Dobyns found that in 1630 Jesuit missions in Paraguay were inundated by a disease that took more than 20 percent of victims. "The whole body was covered by a rash that some called measles and others smallpox, and no one knew what it was."[40] Given the fact that it appeared in the early part of the 1630s, it could have been caused by typhus too. In 1630 the mission of Candelaria, with 7,000 Indian converts, was struck by epidemic infection. By the end of the epidemic, 1,000 Indians fell victim. A settlement of the Caro "was

37 Diego Rodríguez Docampo, "Descripción y relación del estado eclesiástico del obispado de San Francisco de Quito, 1650," in *Relaciones geográficas de Indias, Perú*, ed. Marcos Jiménez de la Espada (Madrid: Atlas, 1965), 3:13; Suzanne Austin Alchon, *Native Society and Disease in Colonial Ecuador* (Cambridge: Cambridge University Press, 1991), p. 61.
38 Suardo, *Diario de Lima*, p. 110; Sebastián de Covarrubias Orozco, *Tesoro de la lengua castellana o española* (Madrid: Editorial Castalia, 1994), refers to *esquinencia* as a disease that begins in the throat; quinsy includes inflammation of the tonsils and formation of pus.
39 Suardo, *Diario*, p. 73.   40 Dobyns, "Andean Epidemic History," p. 509.

ravaged in the early 1630s by disease and famine."[41] The mission of Santo Thomás on the Ibicui, founded in the early 1630s, had a population of 3,000 baptized and 900 schoolchildren. The epidemic that swept through the settlement killed 700 children and 160 adults. San José, also on the Ibicui, was established in 1634. With a population of about 1,200 when epidemic and famine passed through in 1637, "many of its Indians died and most of the survivors were persuaded to flee by their shamans."[42] The Indian settlement of Jesús María had 1,000 young people being indoctrinated when the terrible sickness entered; "with it the people scattered, so that there were hardly any left in the town. Of some 400 boys who used to come to the church, only ten came."[43]

Typhus in the early 1630s seems to have been widespread enough to qualify as a pandemic, rather than an epidemic outbreak. It did appear to afflict residents of highland temperate locales more than those of humid tropical districts, in keeping with the favorite habitat of the carrier, human body lice, in the dirty woolen clothing of its victims. Overall mortality for entire populations seems to have ranged in the 20–25 percent level, similar to known mortality levels for typhus. Contrary to measles and smallpox, European mortality from typhus was probably similar to that of the Amerindians. The periodicity of the major outbreaks came at intervals of about forty years, with the first American pandemic in 1545–46, the second between 1576–91, and the third in 1629–33. As in the case of smallpox, new and very severe epidemics appeared with the completion of a generation.

Yellow Fever in the Late 1640s

Many new migrants to the New World in the seventeenth century came from northern and western Europe, yet the only new Old World pathogen introduced was yellow fever, which was most associated with the expansion of the European slave trade along the coast of Africa. It probably existed in endemic condition in jungle and sylvan form among primates in Africa. In the Americas, marsupials and armadillos can host the disease, and American nonhuman primates are very susceptible. African populations displayed a resistance or tolerance for the virus, indicating that the disease was endemic on that continent. Why did it take the yellow fever virus so long to make the crossing to

41 Hemming, *Red Gold*, p. 261.   42 Ibid., p. 263.   43 Ibid.

the Americas? The answer lies in the very complex etiology of the disease. Yellow fever probably reached America earlier by means of infected individuals, but it did not take firm root. It is spread largely by the bite of the female *Aedes aegypti* mosquito, which is a highly specialized insect that apparently is not native to America and that lives best in close association with *Homo sapiens*. The range of the mosquito is short, and it needs standing water. Water barrels, jugs, even small puddles are ideal for propagation. The female mosquito will not bite when the temperature falls below 17°C, so in temperate climates yellow fever is a problem of the warm months. The symptoms are a sudden illness or lethargy, fever, a slowed pulse, and sometimes the vomiting of blood of at first a light or clear color that becomes darker, getting to be almost black. Hence, at times the sickness was labeled "black vomit." Finally the victim becomes jaundiced, a symptom that most distinguishes yellow fever from other fevers and gives the disease its name.[44]

The first New World yellow fever epidemic, as opposed to a single outbreak among a small number of infected individuals in a restricted area, may have occurred earlier in the colonial era, starting in September 1647. The original focus was the English island of Barbados, which was at the time converting to a plantation-based economy and was in the process of accelerating the importation of slaves from Africa. The population density had reached 200 per square mile, sufficient to sustain a major epidemic. Europeans suffered as great a mortality rate as native Americans during prolonged bouts of yellow fever. The disease lingered in Barbados into 1648 and would recur often enough for it to be called locally the "Barbados distemper." In New England, John Winthrop wrote his son on 6 August 1648 that "Captain Wall came this day from Barbados. Mr. Allen and all our neighbors were safe arrived. Mr. Allen lost but 10 hogs. The plague is *still hot* at Barbados. Mr. Parker, the Minister, and Mr. Longe, who married Captain Hawkins daughter, are dead there."[45] Winthrop of course

---

44 Donald B. Cooper and Kenneth F. Kiple, "Yellow Fever," in *The Cambridge World History of Human Disease*, ed. Kenneth F. Kiple (Cambridge: Cambridge University Press, 1993), pp. 1100–1107; William M. Denevan, "Introduction," in *The Native Population of the Americas in 1492*, ed. William M. Denevan (Madison: University of Wisconsin Press, 1992), p. 5; Woodrow Borah, "Introduction," in *Secret Judgments*, ed. Cook and Lovell, pp. 10–11.

45 John Winthrop, *Winthrop Papers, 1631–1637* (Boston: Massachusetts Historical Society, 1943), 2:384.

refers to yellow fever. During the epidemic, 6,000 on the island died. From Barbados the fever's spread was directly associated with the rapidly expanding communities of its insect vector, the *Aedes aegypti* mosquito.

Yellow fever devastated the island of St. Martin in 1648. From there Bishop Damian López de Haro carried the infection in his body to the island of Margarita, where he died during his pastoral inspection. Severe yellow fever bouts were experienced in the Yucatán peninsula the following year, and in Cuba, St. Kitts, and Guadaloupe in 1649. The first yellow fever pandemic in the New World afflicted most port cities in the Caribbean basin: Campeche in Mexico in 1648, then Mérida in the Yucatán, next Valladolid and its hinterland. There it first hit the European settlements, then entered the Amerindian villages. Yellow fever continued there for about two years. The book *Chilam Balam de Chumayel* provides vivid evidence of the impact of the epidemic on the Yucatán peninsula: "There was bloody vomit and we began to die in the year 1648." The sickness was followed by five years of hunger from 1650 through 1654.[46]

Yellow fever also appeared in San Juan, Puerto Rico, and in Havana, Cuba. In Havana it appears that over a third of the military population succumbed to the sickness. Of an urban population of about 4,670, a total of 562 persons died in 1649, compared to 87 in 1646, 106 in 1647, 134 in 1648, and 148 in 1650. Virtually all the deaths in Havana took place in two months, August and September 1649. About four-fifths of European deaths for the year occurred in these two months but only about half the deaths for Blacks. The difference in mortality between the two groups led to yellow fever being called the "white man's sickness." As late as 1695, mortality was still high among Europeans, for a witness to the epidemic in Santiago de Cuba that year said, "Of those attacked, few escaped with their lives."[47]

46 Miguel Rivera, ed., *Chilam Balam de Chumayel* (Madrid: Historia 16, 1986), p. 117.
47 Kenneth F. Kiple, *The Caribbean Slave: A Biological History* (Cambridge: Cambridge University Press, 1984), pp. 20, 165. See also Woodrow Borah and Sherburne F. Cook, *Essays in Population History*, 3 vols. (Berkeley: University of California Press, 1971–79), 2:115–16; Salvador Brau, *La colonización del Puerto Rico* (San Juan: Instituto de Cultura Puertorriqueña, 1969), pp. 528–29; Henry F. Dobyns, *Their Number Become Thinned: Native American Population Dynamics in Eastern North America* (Knoxville: University of Tennessee Press, 1983), p. 279; and Jorge Leroy y Cassa, *La primera epidemia de fiebre amarilla en la Habana, en 1649* (Havana, 1930).

Yellow fever was found in northern South America, for it reaped its victims in Caribbean Colombia in 1650 and 1651, according to Chandler. In the warmer lowland sectors of Colombia, both yellow fever and malaria ultimately extracted a continuous toll of the human population.[48] But surprisingly yellow fever does not seem to have reached Ecuador in this series, nor did it hit the Brazilian coast. The first epidemic to reach Guayaquil may have been in 1740, with a subsequent one in 1743, although some have argued that Guayaquil's initial yellow fever epidemic was not until 1842.[49]

The contagion was transported on board a ship from Havana to Florida in 1649. In St. Augustine it caused panic and flight, as well as many deaths. The governor of Florida, along with two treasury officials, some military commanders, and missionaries fell.[50] Communications between the infected Caribbean and the Atlantic seaboard were not broken by the contagion, and it could spread everywhere the ships and mosquitoes could be carried, even to the northeastern coasts of North America. Although the malady did not reach New England in the 1640s, it entered New York by 1668, Charleston and Philadelphia in 1690, and finally Boston the following year.

Yellow fever in the late 1640s appears to have been pan-Caribbean, sweeping the Antilles and touching coastal Mexico and the Yucatán, Florida, and the tropical coastal lowlands of South America's north shore. Decades later it exploded beyond the confines of the Caribbean, but at first its range seems to have been limited. Given the large number of slaves being imported into Brazil during these years, plus the endemic nature of yellow fever along part of Africa's coast, scholars have wondered about the absence of the malady in Brazil. Nor did it appear in Guayaquil or in Peru's coastal port of Callao during this period. Perhaps the reason it did not break out in epidemic form at this time in Peru is that the mosquito vector stops laying eggs at 17°C, hence, during most of the year, it would not be present in Callao. But this does not explain its absence in Guayaquil or in the Amazon basin and Brazil. Here other factors must come into play. Perhaps, as Kiple suggests, there was a good chance for survival in populations that had been exposed to endemic sylvan fever, with low rates of mortality, for long periods, as residents of the Amazon must have been. Other viruses may provide some protection against virulent forms of yellow fever, as seems to be true of dengue and Japanese encepha-

48 Chandler, *Health and Slavery*, p. 133.   49 Newson, *Life and Death*, p. 151.
50 Dobyns, *Their Number*, pp. 279–80.

litis.[51] It is also possible that the A. *aegypti* fared poorly against competitors in greater Amazonia, and therefore yellow fever was slow to take root.

LOCALIZED REGIONAL OUTBREAKS: MESOAMERICA

There were only a handful of truly pandemic events during the first fifty years of the seventeenth century, but there were many local outbreaks of disease, several in Mexico alone. Gibson noted the appearance of *cocoliztli* in Xochimilco that began in late 1601 and lasted eight months to June 1602. Several of the most deadly diseases were again found in the central Mexican region in 1604. Measles and mumps, in addition to something that triggered diarrhea, were all noted in the Chimalpahin report for that year, and smallpox could have been present also. Gibson argues that there was a high death rate. In 1613 and 1615–16 smallpox and measles were noted. They were found in Mexico City and were especially prevalent between January and March. Disease was a constant danger in Mexico, where both settlers and natives were attacked.[52] In 1602, an Extremaduran named Alvaro de Paredes wrote to his homeland from Mexico, reporting that he was blessed with six young children. Two years later he had lost two of them, lamenting, "There have been a thousand illnesses and three deaths." He lost two children and a mulatto servant. Young people of European descent in America apparently suffered from Old World disease more than their parents or Old World children who traveled to the New World. Or at least it *seemed* that they did. Altman explains: "Doubtless children born in the Indies were much more susceptible to the epidemic diseases that were ravaging Indian populations than were their parents."[53] Actually, appearances can deceive. Childhood diseases tended to be endemic in the larger, densely populated European cities, and they regularly winnowed the weakest during each passage. During these epidemics, many children suffered mild or subclinical cases, thus acquiring immunity. Furthermore, immunities were constantly reinforced. In America, major

---

51 Cooper and Kiple, "Yellow Fever," p. 1101.
52 Charles Gibson, *The Aztecs Under Spanish Rule. A History of the Indians of the Valley of Mexico, 1519–1810* (Stanford: Stanford University Press, 1964), p. 449; Prem, "Disease Outbreaks in Central Mexico," p. 43.
53 Ida Altman, *Emigrants and Society. Extremadura and America in the Sixteenth Century* (Berkeley: University of California Press, 1989), p. 232.

childhood diseases took place infrequently, at roughly generational intervals. In such cases, almost all young people were susceptible, and many died during an epidemic outbreak. Young people in the New World probably had one survival advantage that in the long run would contribute to population growth. Americans had a more ample and balanced diet than their Old World counterparts.

In 1622 in the Puebla area of central Mexico there were complaints of a "coughing sickness" that led to discomfort and, many times, death. Next year an illness labeled *mal de lutos* broke out. After heavy rains and floods in 1627, illnesses erupted in Mexico City. Measles broke out in 1639, with many deaths. Gibson reports the occurrence in the 1641–42 drought of illness and death and mentions *cocoliztli* and nosebleeds.[54]

Borah and Cook noted famine in 1604 that would have affected the Yucatán, then typhus in 1609, locusts in 1618, smallpox and measles in 1627–31, with four years of bad harvests and famine. These diseases were followed by yellow fever, smallpox, and famine in the period from 1648 to 1656. Disease soon followed resettlement attempts in the Yucatán area. In the period 1612–13 Franciscan missionaries made substantial efforts to concentrate native Americans in towns. Borah and Cook outline the mortality crises of 1627–31 and 1648–57 in the Yucatán peninsula. In the first period, famine, poor crop yields with locusts, and epidemics were experienced.[55]

Lovell found abundant documentation for disease outbreaks in Guatemala. Towns in Chiapas suffered in 1600 "troublesome and long illnesses that have carried away many people." Those suffering most were the natives; many had died, and "because of this there has been starvation."[56] In October 1601 in Cakchiquel communities an epidemic began that attacked the throat; perhaps it was diphtheria. Death could come within two days. Lovell noted what appeared to be localized epidemics in Chiapas in 1607–8 ("the Indians have died of pestilence"), and around 1608 in San Juan Amatitlán "a great many Indians have died during a pestilence."[57] He also found the record of a major bout of an illness characterized by nosebleeds, perhaps typhus, in 1607–8. This was widespread, according to Audiencia officials. The president of the Audiencia, Alonso Criado de Castilla, wrote on 30

54 Prem, "Disease Outbreaks in Central Mexico," p. 43; Gibson, *Aztecs*, p. 450.
55 Borah and Cook, *Essays in Population History*, 2:115–18.
56 Lovell, "Disease in Early Colonial Guatemala," pp. 63, 64, 78, 79.
57 Ibid., p. 64.

November 1608, remarking on the high level of mortality: "With great abruptness, in two or three days, and sometimes almost immediately, these miserable Indians die." Again one of the symptoms was a severe nosebleed that was almost impossible to staunch. No cure seemed to be effective for the malady. The Audiencia president also noted that "typhus was mixed in among some of those stricken."[58] Then, in the valley of Guatemala around 1610 there were "plagues" with many Indian dead. This was followed by the pestilence that appeared in numerous towns in 1612. Again, in 1614 there was "general pestilence" in Santiago de Guatemala. In 1617 "sick Indians" were noted in San Martín Cuchumatán, and in 1618 there were not enough Indians because of the decrease in numbers "by sicknesses and deaths."[59] There was an epidemic in 1623, probably of smallpox, that took primarily children and young people. The city council of Santiago on 9 October 1623 wrote the monarch that many children and young people had died but that "since the beginning of August the sickness that hitherto had been general throughout the country has ceased."[60]

Newson postulates that in the late sixteenth and seventeenth centuries Nicaragua may not have suffered as severely from the ravages of epidemic disease as did Guatemala. Perhaps the population density of Nicaragua was lower than that of Guatemala. She found an epidemic of pneumonic plague described by Audiencia President Alonso Criado de Castilla. He reported that "it did not affect Spaniards but was worst among hispanicized Indians and those who lived in the coldest regions." She did not see evidence of it farther to the south. During the period, "pneumonic plague and typhus were among the most important diseases" to hit Guatemala. She noted that both diseases were more common in cooler zones, so the impact on Nicaragua was less severe.[61]

Andean America

By the seventeenth century several diseases appear to have become endemic in the highlands of western South America. In 1597 there had been measles and pleurisy in Lima. According to Lastres, the century was ushered in by an epidemic at Castrovirreina, a mining

---

58 Ibid., p. 78.   59 Ibid., p. 64.   60 Ibid., p. 79.
61 Newson, *Indian Survival*, pp. 247–48.

center in the highlands to the east of Nazca. Illness was reported in Quito in 1604, then in 1606 *garotillo*, or diphtheria, struck, with many deaths following. In 1606 in Cabana and Huandoval in the central Peruvian Andes there was an epidemic of measles and smallpox that persisted five months.[62] In the community of Aymaya in Upper Peru, 1609 and 1610 were years of higher than normal mortality, with smallpox noted locally. The next bad years in Aymaya were 1620 and 1622.[63] Typhus and measles hit Ecuador in 1611–12, plus scarlet fever, then in 1614 typhus and diphtheria.[64]

In Pocona in 1609 illness swept away 99 percent of the people. Cleric Francisco de Alfaro wrote to Viceroy Marqués de Montesclaros on 29 April 1609 that the repartimiento of Pocona was severely afflicted by an illness the Indians named *"sacha hongo,* which means sickness of the montaña. Because of the humidity the stomach swells up and they become thin and yellowed. Experience has taught us that other repartimientos that are involved in the production of coca have declined and there remain only five boys now alive in the doctrina, but according to the last tribute assessment the repartimiento had 500."[65] Both the eastern and the western slopes of the Andes harbored autochtonous diseases that were long-term killers of both Amerindians and Europeans, and they continue to maim and kill in the twentieth century. The coca fields of the eastern montaña sector, running all the way from Colombia into Bolivia, were ideal sites for Chagas's disease, Carrion's disease, and leishmaniasis. As Gade has pointed out, leish-maniasis was probably the most common of the group. Sandflies are the vector, and they can be either *Phlebotomus* or *Lutzomyia.* Domestic and wild animals act as hosts, and rodents, marsupials, foxes, and dogs can all carry the illness. The disease is produced by protozoa of the genus *Leishmania,* and there are several clinical forms of the disease. The cutaneous form causes skin lesions that tend to be chronic and that may ulcerate. For Andean valleys the *Leishmania braziliensis,* car-

62 Archivo General de Indias, Seville, Lima 33 and Quito 19; Lastres, *Historia de la medicina peruana,* 2:179.

63 Brian Evans, "Death in Aymaya of Upper Peru," in *Secret Judgments,* ed. Cook and Lovell, pp. 150–51.

64 Gualberto Arcos, *Evolución de la medicina en el Ecuador* (Quito: Casa de la Cultura Ecuatoriana, 1979), p. 108; Linda A. Newson, "Old World Epidemics in Early Colonial Ecuador," in *Secret Judgments,* ed. Cook and Lovell, p. 111.

65 Thérèse Bouysse Cassagne, *La identidad aymara. Aproximación histórica (siglo XV, Siglo XVI)* (La Paz: HISBOL, 1987), p. 414.

ried largely by the *Lutzpmyia* sandfly, is the mucocutaneous form, breaking down the membranes of the nose, mouth, and throat, disfiguring, then killing in a process that may take up to four decades. Visceral leishmaniasis develops when the protozoa enter organs, producing intense enlargement of the liver, spleen, and ultimately the abdomen, with diarrhea and anemia. Mortality reaches 75 to 95 percent in untreated cases.[66] The Lima diarist reported that on 2 May 1630, Juan de la Serna died of long-term *berrugas*. He had been in bed for a year and a half "of a painful illness caused at the beginning by some improperly treated *berrugas*."[67] The agent of *berrugas* is a bacterium that is transmitted at night by the bite of the female sandfly *Phlebotomus verrucarum*, whose habitat is in narrow valleys at elevations of 700–2,500 meters. Unfortunately, small mammals act as reservoirs of infection. *Oroya* fever and *verruga peruana* are manifestations of the same disease element. After infection, there are fever, chills, pain in the joints, then a stage marked by anemia, followed ultimately by months or even years of *verrucose* eruptions; some may become painful large nodules prone to bleeding.[68]

In 1614 several epidemics were noted as being possible in the Andean region; they included diphtheria (*garrotillo*) and erysipelas (*erisipela*), with suspicion of scarlet fever (*escarlatina*) and feverish tumors (*fiebres tumores*).[69] Actually "the same streptococci that cause erysipelas (literally red skin) can also cause scarlet fever, giving both diseases a fairly distinctive age pattern." Scarlet fever is normally associated with the young, whereas erysipelas attacks adult populations.[70] Separately, Dobyns argues that Cuzco residents experienced diphtheria in 1614. According to the source, "one's throat swelled and one strangled." So many people died that it was impossible to bury as was normal within the churches, and an outdoor cemetery was set up on the road to Huamanga (Ayacucho) west of the city. The epidemic

66 Daniel W. Gade, "Inca and Colonial Settlements, Coca Cultivation and Endemic Disease in the Tropical Forest," *Journal of Historical Geography* 5(1979):263–79; Marvin J. Allison, "Leishmaniasis," in Kiple, *Cambridge World History*, pp. 832–34.

67 Suardo, *Diario de Lima*, p. 59.

68 Oscar Urteaga-Ballón, "Carrión's Disease," in Kiple, *Cambridge World History*, pp. 631–35.

69 Lastres, *Historia de la medicina peruana*, 2:179.

70 Ann G. Carmichael, "Erysipelas," in Kiple, *Cambridge World History*, pp. 720–21.

continued from May to September, afflicting all elements of the city's population regardless of age, class, or race. As was normal in serious and deadly epidemics, religious processions and prayers were performed to end the scourge without immediate result. Lastres reports scarlet fever may also have been present in Cuzco. The epidemic in Potosí the following year was, according to Dobyns, "probably an episode of the Cuzco contagion."[71]

Smallpox occurred in the Sabana de Bogotá of Colombia in 1621.[72] Friede notes that the population of the mining community of Muzo in Colombia fell from 9,127 people in 1617 to 4,866 in 1629, a period bracketed by epidemics elsewhere; this was a reduction of 46.6 percent in just over a decade. Nearby La Palma during the same period lost inhabitants less precipitously; the tributary population in the same years fell from 1,539 to 1,182. Friede argues that the "wide dispersion of communities or tribes in New Granada, the different climates of their habitants, and their relative isolation, even after the Conquest, were undoubtedly an obstacle to the spread of epidemics."[73]

In Lima typhus took its toll in 1625. Measles recurred in the Lima area in 1628, 1634, and 1635. There was a smallpox outbreak in Huánuco in 1632, and in nearby Chavín de Huantar smallpox was experienced in both 1631 and 1633. To the south, Dobyns reports that the Andean highlands of Argentina were devastated by "measles" and fevers in the period 1634–36.[74] Cuzco was swept in 1644 by disease described as pleurisy and severe cough (catarro). Mortality was significant; the documents state that "many people died." Both measles (here alfombrilla) and diphtheria were noted in Quito in 1645. Just before 1646 an unidentified disease hit the inhabitants of the mining community of Mompox with vigor, and many lives were lost around Popayán. A virulent smallpox epidemic returned to afflict the area of Colombia in 1651.[75]

Thanks to Lima diarists Juan Antonio Suardo, Josephe de Mugu-

---

71 Dobyns, "Andean Epidemic History," p. 509.
72 Villamarin and Villamarin, "Epidemics in the Sabana de Bogotá," p. 114.
73 Juan Friede, "Demographic Changes in the Mining Community of Muzo after the Plague of 1629," Hispanic American Historical Review 47(1967):339–40.
74 Lastres, Historia de la medicina peruana, 2:180; Dobyns, "Andean Epidemic History," p. 510.
75 Lastres, Historia de la medicina peruana, 2:180; Villamarin and Villamarin, "Epidemics in the Sabana de Bogotá," p. 114; Chandler, Health and Slavery, p. 133.

buru, and Muguburu's son Francisco, we have useful firsthand information on sickness in the metropolis from the 1620s to 1694. Suardo, for
example, mentions the case of the death from typhus (27 September
1629) of Licentiate Diego Diez de Tapia, secretary of the University of
San Marcos. On 7 December 1629, there was another case of the
illness. In the morning Jesuit Hieronimo Montesinos, one of the best-
known preachers in Lima, was discovered to have died of typhus. He
had been ill approximately eleven days. So many people came to the
funeral that it was impossible to fit all in the church and monastery,
thus creating excellent conditions for infection of others. Unfortunately, there is no indication if this was part of a widespread epidemic
or isolated cases.[76]

On 14 March 1630, the viceroy ordered that all African slaves that
had just arrived in the port had to stop one league outside Lima's
gates, "the men in one place, the women in another, and the first
thing, by order of his excellency, three physicians had to inspect them
to avoid the illnesses of smallpox and measles that always seemed to
be conveyed with them."[77] It is noteworthy that even as distant as
Lima was to the Caribbean and Brazilian slave centers, by the middle
of the seventeenth century the human traffic had come to be associated with the importation of disease. Fresh cases of measles and smallpox could do great damage to Amerindians especially, but the virulent
strains wrought havoc on the creole population too. In Lima, as
elsewhere in the Indies, quarantine was widely practiced to avoid
contagion. Unfortunately, it was rarely successful.

In February through March of 1645, measles and diphtheria struck
Ecuador. Morbidity seems to have been high; of ninety boys in the
San Luis Seminary, eighty-seven fell sick, and natives in the countryside fell ill and died in large numbers. Deaths from measles and
diphtheria continued, although at lower levels until smallpox and
measles combined took lives. Town council members of Quito indicate
that perhaps 100,000 people succumbed to the compound epidemic in
1648. Eastern lowland districts were especially hard hit. Diego
Rodríguez Docampo compared its ravages, extending into 1649, to the
devastating series of 1587–88.[78]

76 Suardo, Diario de Lima, pp. 23, 34.
77 Ibid., p. 51.
78 Marcos Jiménez de la Espada, ed., Relaciones geográficas de Indias, Peru, 3 vols.
    (Madrid: Atlas, 1965), 3:70; Suzanne Austin Alchon, Native Society and Dis-

The Upper Amazon Basin

Spanish intentions to settle the Upper Amazon basin in the sixteenth century ended in failure in spite of a handful of dramatic attempts. By the seventeenth century there were renewed Spanish efforts, on the one hand, to Christianize the "barbarian" peoples of the jungle and, on the other, to prevent the Portuguese from making a territorial claim based on effective land settlement. The focus of expeditions sent out from Peru tended to be in the Maynas territory, in the lower Morona and Pastaza river systems, to the north of the great Marañón River and immediately following the rapids of the Pongo de Manseriche. There were two major sixteenth-century expeditions into the region from Peru, and there was continuous although limited contact with Spanish settlers from the Upper Marañón dating from the 1580s. Viceroy Montesclaros organized Maynas settlement from the Spanish town of Loja in 1613. That rather small frontier outpost became the headquarters for the preparation and provisioning of excursions downriver. The military expeditions led to forcible and uneasy settlement of native peoples in the area. Although the evidence is sparse, David Sweet surmises that European diseases arrived before 1619.[79] Indeed, the epidemic series ending in the early 1590s was particularly devastating to peoples in the eastern montaña of Ecuador. The focus of European settlement among the Maynas was at the frontier post of Borja, and when the encomenderos received the first Indian grants there in 1619, there were about 700 tributaries and a total population of perhaps 3,500. In the initial years there was much movement of natives in and out of Borja, resulting in an unstable population. Even in the absence of initial epidemics, the native Amazonians at Borja failed to reproduce successfully. Perhaps nutritional deficiencies and the new regulated regime took the spirit out of many of them, as Jackson has argued recently for the missions of northwest New Spain later in the century. Sweet also noted a typical "pine away and die" syndrome characteristic of many mission settlements. Furthermore, there was a serious uprising against encomenderos in 1635, in which some 1,000 Maynas fighters joined forces against the outsiders. By the

ease in Colonial Ecuador (Cambridge: Cambridge University Press, 1991), p. 62.
79 David G. Sweet, "The Population of the Upper Amazon Valley, Seventeenth and Eighteenth Centuries," M.A. thesis (Madison: University of Wisconsin, 1969), p. 13.

time the rebellion was subdued by soldiers and Jesuits, only 400 tributaries and a total of 1,600 persons remained at Borja in 1638. Contemporaries argued that the less than twenty-year decline of more than 75
percent of the native population was caused by rebellion, illnesses, or
internecine warfare "in that order of importance."[80] Furthermore, a
terrible outbreak of smallpox occurred in 1642, and almost all who
succumbed were children.

Francisco de Figueroa, a Jesuit missionary in the Maynas, chronicled
his experiences. Shortly after his arrival in Borja, he was among those
to care for natives who had been infected by the smallpox.[81] As he
was finishing his history of the mission in 1661, there were only 200
Maynas tributaries left. He wrote that they had died as the consequence of "disease, warfare and non-reproduction," in that sequence.[82]
In 1660–61, some 340 fugitives and pagans were captured and brought
back to Borja; unfortunately, "more than that number died of measles
and valley sickness."[83] Figueroa lamented in 1661: "It has been the
experience of these Indians that when the Light of Heaven bursts into
their miserable huts it is followed forthwith by the shadowy horrors of
plague and decimation." Already at the time he wrote his account of
the Maynas and nearby tribal groups, at least half had died "with their
humors altered so as to produce deathly illness, by the detonations of
the harquebus, the smell of powder and the shock of bullets."[84] Conquest by disease continued in the Amazon basin into the seventeenth
century.

COASTAL BRAZIL

Devastation of Brazil's coastal peoples persisted into the seventeenth
century. (See Table 5.3.) Accelerating slave trade with Africa probably
influenced the timing and virulence of epidemic outbreaks. During the
early seventeenth century, shipments of slaves ranged from 4,000 to

---

80 Francisco de Figueroa, *Relación de las misiones de la Compañía de Jesús en el país
de los Maynas* (Madrid, 1904), pp. 15–16; Sweet, "Population of the Upper
Amazon," p. 13; Robert H. Jackson, *Indian Population Decline. The Missions of
Northwestern New Spain, 1687–1840* (Albuquerque: University of New Mexico
Press, 1994).
81 Figueroa, *Relación de las misiones*, pp. 25, 34.
82 Ibid., pp. 15–16, 25, 34.   83 Ibid., p. 22.
84 Sweet, "Population of the Upper Amazon," pp. 23–24; Figueroa, *Relación de
las misiones*, pp. 166–67, 182, 184.

Table 5.3. *Epidemics along the*
Brazilian coast, 1600–1650

Date	Disease
1611	Smallpox, São Paulo (?)
1613	Smallpox, Pernambuco
1616	Smallpox, Northeast
1621–23	Smallpox, Northeast
1626	Smallpox, Bahia
1630	Epidemic and famine
1637	Epidemic and famine
1641	Smallpox, Northeast
1642	Smallpox
1644	Smallpox, Maranhao
1645	Catarrhs (influenza?)

7,000 people yearly. Smallpox blanketed Pernambuco and the northeast from 1621 to 1623. The link with the African slave trade was strong, and for the first time municipal officials in Pernambuco imposed quarantine for arriving slaves. Disease along the coast of Africa was widespread and serious in the mid-1620s. Angola, a primary supply area for Brazil at the time, was beset by drought and a major smallpox epidemic in 1625–28. Many slave ships sailed out of Luanda, Angola's principal port city, in the mid-1620s. There was extraordinarily high slave mortality during the crossings, yet individuals infected with smallpox were landed at Salvador.[85]

Dutch control over coastal Maranhao did little or nothing to change the level of native mortality. Indeed, an epidemic of smallpox is reported from late 1641 to early 1642. Beginning in Paraíba and Itamaraca, it swept northward to engulf Rio Grande and Ceará. It "raged so violently among the Indians that entire aldeas were almost totally extinguished. The survivors retreated into the forests since they

---

85 Dauril Alden and Joseph C. Miller, "Unwanted Cargoes: The Origin and Dissemination of Smallpox via the Slave Trade, c. 1560–1830," in *The African Exchange: Toward a Biological History of Black People*, ed. Kenneth F. Kiple (Durham: Duke University Press, 1987), p. 201; see also Joseph C. Miller, "The Significance of Drought, Disease and Famine in the Agriculturally Marginal Zones of West-Central Africa," *Journal of African History* 23 (1982):17–61.

no longer dared to remain in their homes."[86] Alden and Miller, after careful archival research, found that in 1644, "smallpox caused extensive losses among the Indian villages of Maranhao."[87] Antonio Teixeira de Mello reported to the king on 14 March 1645 that the Dutch "brought not only war but also plague. For they brought with them Indians with smallpox, which is the plague of that land. They thus killed the majority of the best people in our Indian aldeas and almost all the settlers' slaves."[88]

NORTH AMERICA

According to a series of reports to the Spanish monarch filed by Franciscan missionaries in La Florida, illness that killed half the nearby Guale and Timucuan Indians lingered from 1613 to 1617. On 17 January 1617, the Franciscans wrote to the king, complaining that they had found that in the past four years, "half the Indians have disappeared as a result of the great sicknesses and contagious epidemics that they have suffered." Just as in the case of the Jesuit Francisco de Figueroa in the Maynas missions of the Upper Amazon, the Franciscan friars in Florida found satisfaction, in spite of the tremendous loss of human life, that at least "these deaths have taken great harvests of souls for heaven. There remain alive almost eight thousand Christians."[89] Dobyns identified the sickness as a possible plague outbreak, although the evidence is inconclusive. The Franciscan letter is more suggestive of a series of discrete illnesses during the four years. *Peste* (plague) may have been one element, although as Dobyns also notes, the word is inexact, meaning either the plague, or more broadly, any epidemic contagion. Without precise description of symptoms, it is impossible to say what diseases passed through the region in 1613–17.

Reff's analysis of the Jesuit letters suggests that smallpox had become endemic in the southwestern borderlands by the early seventeenth century. Measles also recurred frequently. Furthermore, bubonic plague was reported among the Hopis in a 1613–16 epidemic. Measles hit the Pueblo region around 1635, and a smallpox epidemic followed

---

86 Hemming, *Red Gold*, p. 293.
87 Alden and Miller, "Unwanted Cargoes," p. 202.
88 Hemming, *Red Gold*, p. 293.
89 Luis Gerónimo de Oré, *Relación histórica de la Florida, escrito en el siglo XII*, 2 vols. (Madrid, 1931–33), 2:41.

Table 5.4. *Disease chronology of*
northwestern Mexico, 1601–1653

1601–2	Smallpox, measles, typhus
1606–7	Smallpox, measles
1612–15	Typhus, smallpox (?)
1616–17	Measles and/or smallpox
1619–20	Various ailments
1623–25	Smallpox, typhus, pneumonia
1636–41	Smallpox and "other maladies"
1645–47	"Malicious fevers" (malaria?)
1652–53	Smallpox and "other maladies"

in 1641. (See Table 5.4.) Missionary Juan de Prado in 1638 wrote of the devastation caused by smallpox among the Pueblo peoples. "The people that may be counted today in these settlements will total 40,000, or a little less, for although there must have been more than 60,000 baptized, today those conversions are diminished to that extent on account of the very active prevalence of smallpox."[90]

The French came relatively late to the Mississippi basin and arrived in small numbers. What they lacked in force they made up for by their great mobility in the interior, both the trappers and fur traders, as well as the missionaries. Their explosive force in the early to middle seventeenth century reminds one of the militant crusading Christian fervor of the sixteenth-century Spanish missionaries. The great explorers Louis Jolliet and René-Robert Cavelier de La Salle expanded French geographical knowledge and influence down the Mississippi, then up its tributaries, especially to the west toward lands claimed by the Spanish.[91]

More permanent French settlement took place with Champlain's

90 Ann F. Ramenofsky, *Vectors of Death: The Archeology of European Contact* (Albuquerque: University of New Mexico Press, 1987), p. 133; Daniel T. Reff, *Disease, Depopulation, and Culture Change in Northwestern New Spain, 1518–1764* (Salt Lake City: University of Utah Press, 1991), pp. 169–72. Jackson, *Indian Population Decline*, provides excellent data for epidemics in the region from the late seventeenth century but does not enter arguments on disease prior to the dates for which he has solid mission records.

91 Thornton, *American Indian Holocaust*, p. 76.

foundation on the Isle de Saint Croix, followed by the establishment
of Quebec in 1608. Henry Hudson's 1609 voyage up the river that was
later named after him was followed in the next five years by four Dutch
ships trading for pelts and bringing foreign pathogens. In addition to
French efforts in the St. Lawrence area and Quebec in 1608, the
English founded Jamestown to the south in 1607, and Dutch traders
set up Fort Nassau near Albany in 1614. The English settlement at
Plymouth in 1619 resulted in continuous contact and regular written
accounts of much of what happened. Thereafter, the historical record,
in spite of the difficulty of accurate disease diagnosis, is almost continuous. Traveling along with trade goods went diseases.

Epidemics were regularly introduced into New France. As Gelfand
has noted, the annual fleet to Quebec brought not only needed supplies; it also brought passengers with "malignant fevers," perhaps typhoid, typhus, and influenza. Both Huron and Iroquois came to trade
at Quebec shortly after it was established in 1608. When French
contact was made, the Huron were settled in about 28 palisaded
villages in a 340-square-mile tract of land in present Ontario, with a
total population of perhaps 20,000 to 35,000. They were agriculturalists, growing corn, pumpkins, squash, beans, and other crops. They
supplemented their diets by hunting and fishing. Villages might include 100 long houses, each containing a number of extended family
members. When the French arrived in force at the beginning of
the seventeenth century, the Huron were fighting with the Iroquois,
especially the Seneca. The French quickly saw a chance for profit and
established posts to trade European weapons and iron tools for Indian
furs, thus exacerbating already-existing intertribal warfare. The cross
was introduced too. The missionary settlement of Sainte Marie in
1639 was to be an important step in the conversion of the Huron. Just
as settlement was becoming more pronounced, and native peoples
were increasingly entering into close personal contact with the outsiders, disaster struck. Between 1634 and 1640 a series of epidemics
broke out, with smallpox being a principal component. When the
illness started in 1636, "terror was universal. The contagion increased
as autumn advanced; and when winter came, its ravages were appalling. The season of the Huron festivity was turned to a season of
mourning; and such was the despondency and dismay, that suicides
became frequent. . . . Everywhere was heard the wail of the sick and
dying children; and on or under the platforms at the sides of the

house crouched squalid men and women, in all stages of distemper."[92] The Jesuits came to play a special role in the settlement of Canada, where many natives soon believed that they had curative powers. Certainly the Jesuits assisted many of those who fell ill during the major epidemics, providing food, water and firewood, as well as European medicines such as raisins, sugar, prunes, lemon rinds, and perhaps theriac and senna. Bleeding was also tried, with Jesuit Simon Baron actively practicing the art among the Huron in 1636–37. The fact that the Jesuits seemed to thrive while the natives continued to die had a profound emotional impact. Axtell concludes "initially, in the disorienting chaos and sweeping mortality of the first wave of epidemics, they feared the black-robed strangers as 'demons' and 'sorcerers' who had spawned the diseases to conquer them."[93] One ceremony the Huron quickly associated with the Jesuits was baptism, with the appropriate movements, incantations, and sprinkling of water. It was not surprising that just as in Brazil, the natives soon concluded that "the suspicious act of baptism caused the death of their relatives and loved ones." Yet enough did recover after baptism so that by the time of the 1636–37 Huron epidemic, one aspiring shaman used for a cure a "mysterious water with which he sprinkled the sick."[94]

Smallpox was reported again in 1639 in the St. Lawrence valley, and in 1640 among the Huron. Gelfand believes that smallpox arrived in Quebec in 1640 with the new fleet, which was carrying religious nursing sisters for the Hôtel-Dieu.[95] Major new smallpox epidemics swept across Canada in 1649–50, according to Grumet, and many more epidemics were introduced in the eighteenth century. By 1640 there were only 10,000 Huron left out of an estimated 20,000 to 35,000 in the early 1600s, and warfare with their Iroquois enemies in the 1640s almost completely wiped out the remaining members of the tribe.[96] The Iroquois themselves suffered a similar fate two decades

92 Toby Gelfand, "Medicine in New France," in *Medicine in the New World: New Spain, New France, and New England*, ed. Ronald L. Numbers (Knoxville: University of Tennessee Press, 1987), p. 77; Thornton, *American Indian Holocaust*, p. 74; Francis Parkman, *The Jesuits in North America in the Seventeeth Century* (Boston: New Library, 1909), p. 87.
93 James Axtell, *The Invasion Within: The Contest of Cultures in Colonial North America* (New York: Oxford University Press, 1985), pp. 86, 97.
94 Ibid., p. 123.   95 Gelfand, "Medicine in New France," p. 77.
96 Robert Steven Grumet, " 'How Strangely They Have Decreast by the Hand of God': An Historic Epidemiology of the Upper Delawaran People." Paper

Table 5.5. *Northeastern epidemics in the*
seventeenth century

New England	New York	New France
1612–13		
1616		
1617		
1633–34	1634	1634–41
1649	1649	1647

later when one of the smallpox epidemics of the early 1660s "wrought sad havoc in their villages and has carried off many men, besides great numbers of women and children; and as a result their villages are nearly deserted, and their fields are only half-tilled."[97] (See Table 5.5.)

Smallpox visited New England regularly following the 1630s. Sherburne F. Cook concluded that smallpox after 1630–40 "was never absent among the populations of eastern North America." Indeed, "at intervals it flared into epidemic proportions as it reached new Indian tribes, or attacked the non-immune younger generations in older territory."[98] Smallpox was introduced into the New England region earlier even than English settlement. Yet the spread of smallpox among the aboriginal population was accentuated with the massive Puritan migration to New England in 1630. Francis Higginson reported that on the Atlantic crossing both his young children came down with the pox, and one died. Others on the ship fell ill too, but in the words of Higginson, "thanks be to God none dyed of it but my own childe." Another colonist wrote of his passage in March 1631 that "we ware wondurfule seick as we cam at sea withe the small Poxe."

William Bradford reported that an "infectious fever" afflicted the Plymouth settlers in 1633 and carried away twenty of them. But the

presented at the 1983 Native American Historic Epidemiology Conference, the Newberry Library, Chicago, pp. 6–15; Thornton, *American Indian Holocaust*, pp. 73–74.

97 Thornton, *American Indian Holocaust*, p. 74; John Duffy, "Smallpox and the Indians in the American Colonies," *Bulletin of the History of Medicine* 25(1951):329.

98 Sherburne F. Cook, "The Significance of Disease in the Extinction of the New England Indian," *Human Biology* 45(1973):493.

sickness was much worse for surrounding natives, for in his words, "this disease also swept away many of the Indians from all the places near adjoining."[99] In the winter months of 1633–34, Bradford noted that a group of a thousand Indians up the Connecticut River valley, living in a palisaded village, were visited by three or four Dutch traders. Soon the people came down "with a great sickness and such a mortality that of a thousand, above nine and a half hundred of them died, and many of them did rot above ground for want of burial." That same spring, the Indians living near the Plymouth trading house of Windsor, also in the Connecticut valley, "fell sick of the small pox, and died most miserably; for a sorer disease cannot befall them, they fear it more than the plague." In the century following the initial introduction of the disease, wave after wave of smallpox had afflicted the Americas, taking its deadly toll of native peoples. The suffering that the disease extracted was just as severe in 1634 as it had been in 1518. The vivid and excruciating descriptions of smallpox that the Aztecs gave to Friar Bernardino de Sahagún are very similar to those recorded by Governor William Bradford for the natives of New England, who suffered a parallel disaster. Bradford's description mirrors, in nearly all aspects, that of the Aztec encounter with the dreaded disease:

> For usually they that have this disease have them in abundance, and for want of bedding and linen and other helps they fall into a lamentable condition as they lie on their hard mats, the pox breaking and mattering and running one into another, their skin cleaving by reason thereof to the mats they lie on. When they turn them, a whole side will flay off at once as it were, and they will be all of a gore blood, most fearful to behold. And then being very sore, what with cold and other distempers, they die like rotten sheep. The condition of this people was so lamentable and they fell down so generally of this disease as they were in the end not able to help one another, no not to make a fire nor to fetch a little water to drink, nor any to bury the dead. But would strive as long as they could, and when they could procure no other means to make a fire, they would burn the wooden trays and dishes they ate their meat in, and their very bows and arrows. And some would crawl out on all fours to get a little

99 William Bradford, *Of Plymouth Plantation, 1620–1647* (New York: Alfred A. Knopf, 1952), p. 260.

water, and sometimes die by the way and not be able to get in again.[100]

Mortality was negligible among the Europeans, except for small children who had not yet been exposed to the virus. On 12 December 1634, John Winthrop wrote to his son that a boy had "died of the small pox which are very rife at Newtowne."[101]

Grumet found evidence for a northeastern influenza outbreak in 1646. Another epidemic, perhaps a continuation of influenza, passed through New England in 1647. John Winthrop wrote in April of that year that "an epidemical sickness was through the country among Indians and English, French and Dutch. It took them like a cold, and a light fever with it. Such as bled or used cooling drinks died; those who took comfortable things, for most part recovered, and that in few days." Winthrop reported that virtually all families faced the sickness, and he noted that convalescence was slow. The actual mortality rate for the Europeans was low: "Few died, not above forty or fifty in the Massachusetts, and near as many at Connecticut." In all, at least twenty-four epidemics were recorded in a broadly defined "northeast" in the seventeenth century. By the late sixteenth or early seventeenth century, the northeast "constituted a single disease interaction sphere." Ramenofsky concluded that "the 1634–1641 epidemic may have originated in New England, spreading north and west. Recent archaeological evidence for the area confirms the historical data that native Americans were dying rapidly. Almost all past estimates of population size for the native peoples of northeastern North America have been based on peoples already under epidemic pressures."[102]

ASSESSMENT

Large parcels of land were opened over vast stretches of the Americas by the spread of disease. Dobyns quite appropriately calls the process the "winnowing of the land." Foreign latecomers often took advantage of what seemed to be free and unclaimed virgin fields opened by

100 Ibid., pp. 270–71.
101 John Duffy, Epidemics in Colonial America (Baton Rouge: Louisiana State University Press, 1953), pp. 43–44.
102 Grumet, "Epidemiology," pp. 6–7; John Winthrop, Winthrop Papers, 1631–1637, 2 vols. (Boston: Massachusetts Historical Society, 1943), 2:362; Ramenofsky, Vectors of Death, pp. 42–71.

Divine Providence for the "chosen people," the harbingers of a new civilization. The Christian justification for the process is most force-fully put by the early Puritan settlers of New England, who entered territories long claimed by the Spanish and clearly already inhabited by others. They saw the remains of native Americans who succumbed to the ravages of the 1616–19 epidemic of plague, and they witnessed the agony of Massasoit and his kin when they suffered losses from foreign sicknesses. Squanto, who had been to England and knew English well, and who was helpful to the Plymouth settlers, discovered on his return to his homeland in 1618 that he was "the sole survivor of his tribe, wiped out in the pestilence of 1618."[103]

John Cotton in 1630 provided the rationalization for the English settlers. Citing the Old Testament (Genesis 1:28), Cotton noted that God had told Adam and Noah to "come and inhabit . . . where there is a vacant place," without purchase or permission.[104] In similar vein, John Winthrop, a lawyer and first governor of the Massachusetts Bay Colony, wrote a discourse on "Diverse objections which have been made against this Plantation, with their answers and Resolutions," around 1629. The chief objection to the settlement was that the land was already occupied. But because the aboriginal residents did not fence lands and they had plenty, "we may lawfully take the rest, there being more than enough for them and us." Furthermore, Winthrop argued that they would benefit from the European settlers, and most important "for our purposes here, God hath consumed the natives with a great plague in those parts, so as there be few inhabitants left."[105] On 3 January 1634, he wrote to John Endicott to rationalize the survival of the Europeans and the demise of the Indians: "If God were not pleased with our inheriting these parts, why did he drive out the natives before us? and why dothe he still make roome for us, by deminishinge them as we increase?"[106] More forcefully, writing on 22 May, Winthrop justified the new demographic disaster that had just reduced the local natives: "For the natives, they are neere all dead of small Poxe, so as the Lord hathe cleared our title to what we possess."[107]

Other Englishmen concurred with the analysis of Governor Win-throp. William Wood, who referred to the smallpox epidemic of 1633

103 Bradford, *Plymouth Plantation*, ftn., p. 81; Ramenofsky, *Vectors of Death*.
104 Dobyns, *Their Number*, p. 45.   105 Winthrop, *Winthrop Papers*, 1:312.
106 Vaughan, *New England Frontier*, p. 104; Winthrop, *Winthrop Papers*, 3:149.
107 Winthrop, *Winthrop Papers*, 3:167.

in his *New England's Prospect* (1634), wrote that the "Lord put an end to this quarrel by smiting them with smallpox. . . . Thus did the Lord allay their quarrelsome spirit and make room for the following part of his army."[108]

It is informative to contrast the Spanish evaluation of the demise of the native Americans with that of the English. The Spanish largely bemoaned the disappearance of the Amerindian. No one better exemplifies the Iberian attitude than Bartolomé de las Casas, who spent most of his adult life writing and speaking to protect the natives. Even settlers, and some of the worst, such as Pedro de Alvarado, soon recognized that they had too much to lose and much to gain if the native Americans survived to till their fields, to work in their mines, to labor in their households.

The attitude of the English was less concerned with either the material or the spiritual welfare of their Amerindian neighbors. In fact, the Indians stood in the way of what many English Puritan colonists believed to be their divinely inspired attempt to create God's city in the wilderness. If the native Americans perished, it was part of divine will to open up lands for God's "elect." Although the English knew nothing of the germ theory of the spread of disease, they did not reject in some cases the consequences of the introduction of sicknesses that struck the Indians and left the English free, unscathed, ready to take the land of their Indian neighbors. The English did understand quarantine and could have attempted to block the passage of smallpox; the Spanish and Portuguese both did try, albeit unsuccessfully in the sixteenth century, to protect the natives. But the English not only failed to quarantine; they unabashedly welcomed the providential removal of the original inhabitants of the land so that they would be free to found their own communities and prosper without being troubled by people they regarded as savages.

108 William H. McNeill, *Plagues and Peoples* (Garden City, NY: Anchor Doubleday, 1976), pp. 186, 310. See also Arno Karlen, *Man and Microbes, Disease and Plagues in History and Modern Times* (New York: G. P. Putnam's Sons, 1995), p. 104.

CONCLUSION

The Indians . . . affirm, that before the arrival of the Christians, and before the small pox broke out amongst them, they were ten times as numerous as they now are, and that their population had been melted down by this disease.

Adriaen Van der Donck, New Netherland, 1656

You will do well to try to innoculate the Indians by means of blankets as well as to try every other method that can serve to extirpate this execrable race.

Sir Jeffrey Amherst, 1763

The anonymous 1528 Nahuatl account of Tlatelolco depicts the native view of the vicious force Spaniards employed to secure subjugation of Amerindian peoples: "They fed the Keeper of the Black House, along with several others, to their dogs. And three wise men of Ehecatl, from Tezcoco, were devoured by the dogs. They had come only to surrender."[1] Bartolomé de las Casas, Girolamo Benzoni, and many of their contemporaries vividly pointed out that conquest took place by regular and often excessive use of the sword, the lance, the cannon, and the arquebus. The Europeans exerted force, and it was brutal, as they first established a beachhead and then moved into the hinterland to set up permanent settlements in densely populated districts. The horses, armor, gunpowder, ships, and attack dogs were applied in combination to ensure survival and domination by the outsiders. Some native groups joined the foreigners, hoping to right

1 Miguel León-Portilla, ed., *Broken Spears: The Aztec Account of the Conquest of Mexico* (Boston: Beacon Press, 1992), p. 144.

past wrongs or to become part of a new ruling class. Military force, often employed with excessive zeal and with disastrous consequences for New World peoples, was a key factor in the European conquest of America. But even more important as an ally for the foreigners was epidemic disease.

The first smallpox pandemic that swept the Caribbean and Mesoamerica and turned the native world upside down was vividly etched into the minds of the Amerindians. The impact of this scourge was immediate, and its memory lingered long in the minds of those who witnessed its destructive course. One Nahuatl text relates that "while the Spaniards were in Tlaxcala, a great plague broke out here in Tenochtitlan. It began to spread during the thirteenth month [30 September through 19 October 1520] and lasted for seventy days, striking everywhere in the city, and killing a vast number of our people." The witness bemoaned in excruciating detail the pain and suffering the disease inflicted on its victims:

> Sores erupted on our faces, our breasts, our bellies; we were covered with agonizing sores from head to foot. The illness was so dreadful that no one could walk or move. The sick were so utterly helpless that they could only lie on their beds like corpses, unable to move their limbs or even their heads. They could not lie face down or roll from one side to the other. If they did move their bodies, they screamed with pain.

As is so often the case when an epidemic sweeps through an area with most of the population falling ill simultaneously, almost no one remained to provide water and food for those infected and convalescing. Nor was anyone available to tend to the normal agricultural tasks. The immediate consequence was excessive mortality, followed by a year of famine and starvation, and a subsequent passage of another killer pandemic, exacerbating mortality. Again, the native voice poignantly depicts scenes reminiscent of Dante's inferno: "A great many died from this plague, and many others died of hunger. They could not get up to search for food, and everyone else was too sick to care for them, so they starved to death in their beds."[2] The native artist who so well visually depicted the first smallpox epidemic to lash central

---

2 W. George Lovell, " 'Heavy Shadows and Black Night': Disease and Depopulation in Colonial Spanish America," in *Annals of the Association of American Geographers* 82(1992):429.

Mexico (see Figure 2.1, *Codex Florentino*) portrayed five Mesoamericans with fully developed smallpox. Three lie on mats with their eyes closed. Their bodies are completely covered by the characteristic pustules. Another seems to turn and appears to be in agony. The fifth, perhaps a survivor, is seated and is being assisted to ease the pain.

The Mesoamerican vision of the vanquished as they suffered from the dreadful first smallpox crisis is echoed in the Andean world. Native chronicler Juan de Santa Cruz Pachacuti Yamque, born in the highlands between Cuzco and Lake Titicaca, remembered in the first years of the seventeenth century the tragic death of Huayna Capac and the fall of his people at the hands of the outsiders. Although written long after the events, his description mirrors the collapse of the aboriginal world. The account of the death of the last Inca begins as the ruler was returning to Quito after northern conquests. As he marched toward the coast with his army,

> at midnight he saw his headquarters clearly surrounded by a thousand million men, and they did not know them nor understand who they were. At this they say that he said they were the souls of the living, that God had given a sign signifying that so many had to die in the pestilence. The souls said that they came against the Inca, from which the Inca understood that it [pestilence] was his enemy.

The ruler returned to Quito with his troops to conduct the traditional religious ceremonies of the festival of Capacraimi. One day, at mealtime,

> a messenger in a black cloak arrived. He [like Judas] reverently kissed the Inca, and gave the Inca a *putti*, or small covered box with a lock. The Inca ordered the same Indian to open it; he said forgive me, but the Creator ordered him that only the Inca open it. The Inca, seeing the truth, opened the small box, and from it left, as butterflies or *papelillos* [bits of paper, an alternate meaning is pharmaceutical prescriptions], flying or dispersing until they disappeared. It was the pestilence of measles [*sic*], and within two days the general Mihacnacamayta with many other captains died, all their faces covered with scabs.

Fearing the worst, the Inca ordered the building of a stone structure and entered it, hoping to escape sickness in this way. But even the stones erected to seal the house were not enough to keep the conta-

gion out, and the Inca fell ill, and died. After eight days, the chronicler, Santa Cruz Pachacuti, relates, his half-decomposed body was
removed, embalmed, and taken to Cuzco for the traditional ceremonies.[3]

Native author Felipe Guaman Poma de Ayala also rendered in pen
and ink the historical events of the Andean region. Writing between
1567 and 1615,[4] he related:

> They say that by the devil's luck he [Guayna Capac] learned that
> the Spaniards would come to rule. . . . And he died in the city of
> Tumi [Pampa] of a pestilence of measles, smallpox. And in fear
> of death he fled from the contact of men and placed himself
> within a stone structure. And within it he died without others
> knowing of it, but he earlier had ordered that when he died his
> death should not be announced. And they said that he was alive,
> and took him to Cuzco as if his body were alive because he did
> not want the Indians to rise up.[5]

The native chronicler also relates that the Inca's principal wife, Coya
Raua Ocllo, died at the time.[6] Guaman Poma's drawing of the embalmed *huaca*, or mummy bundle, of Huayna Capac as it appeared to
those who saw it carried on a litter across the Andes toward the
imperial capital of Cuzco is a powerful native testament to death by
disease. (See Figure 2.3.) Guaman Poma depicted, along with the Inca
on the litter, two others – a woman and a boy. The eyes of all three
are closed, indicating that the wife of the Inca, as well as his son
Ninan Cuyoche, who according to various texts had died of the same
illness, was also mummified and traveled with him. Guaman Poma
stressed that the victory of the outsiders was made possible by the
division and internal warfare that resulted from the death of Huayna
Capac. The litter traveled southward on the royal highway, roughly
from Quito to Jauja and on to Cuzco. Those who had embalmed the

---

3 Juan Santa Cruz Pachacuti Yamque, *Historia de los Incas* (Lima: Imprenta
  Sanmartí, 1927), pp. 215–16.
4 Raúl Porras Barrenechea, *Los cronistas del Perú (1528–1650) y otros ensayos*, ed.
  Franklin Pease G.Y. (Lima: Banco de Crédito, 1986), p. 616.
5 Felipe Guaman Poma de Ayala, *El primer nueva corónica y buen gobierno*, ed.
  John V. Murra and Rolena Adorno, 3 vols. (México: Siglo Veintiuno, 1980),
  1:93.
6 Ibid., 1:119.

bodies, as well as the litter bearers, must have had ample close physical contact to infect or reinfect with the smallpox virus much of the central Andes.[7]

The sword, important as it was in the destruction of native-American political units and in the creation of colonial empires, paled as the real killer that made European victory possible. It was the fourth horseman of the Apocalypse, invisible germs and vermin, the viruses and bacteria, that killed Amerindians by the hundreds of thousands and millions. Disease was the true weapon of Santiago Matamoros (*Mataindios*), not the sword carried in the Spanish conqueror's hand.[8] The tragic collapse of Amerindian America began a scant half millennium ago. In some regions – the islands of Hispaniola, Cuba, and Puerto Rico, for example – destruction was virtually complete. But in other places in the Americas, native peoples survived and by the late nineteenth century were increasing in numbers. The westward sailing route to the Orient that was opened by Christopher Columbus brought the peoples of a hemisphere hitherto largely isolated into regular and intimate relations with the inhabitants of the great land masses of the ancient world. The consequences of that link between the Old and New Worlds were complex and persisted in both positive and negative senses. The exchange of plants and animals, the dissemination of religious and political philosophies, the evolution of a modern economic order, the rapid adoption of new technologies, the biological mingling of *Homo sapiens*, the spread of alien diseases – all flowed inexorably from the global trade network created by the heirs of Columbus.

The Europeans contributed many new and serious diseases to the American environment. Smallpox and measles were two of the most deadly for the native Americans. Both affected Old World peoples, but both had been largely endemic in Europe and were mostly childhood diseases there. The ports of Andalusia, from which most of the early voyages initiated, were hit by epidemic after epidemic. Most

---

7 Ibid., 2:350–51.
8 Saint James the Greater, or Santiago, is associated with the long Christian reconquest of the Iberian peninsula from the Moors. In art he is usually depicted with sword in hand, mounted on a white horse whose hooves trample the defeated infidel. At times in the Americas Santiago Matamoros, or the Moor Slayer, is painted with fallen Amerindians. See Mickey Abel-Turby, "The New World Augustinians and Franciscans in Philosophical Opposition: The Visual Statement," *Colonial Latin American Review* 5(1996):7–23.

sailors were old enough to have contracted either smallpox or measles before they first sailed. Hence, it would be several years before there would be someone who had not had the disease to become infected and transmit it on board to another as in a chain, until the deadly cargo was unwittingly unloaded on virgin New World shores. It would be otherwise with influenza, which in its various forms mutated with facility; one experience with influenza afforded the individual no significant protection in a later epidemic. But smallpox, measles, and influenza are only three, albeit among the most communicable, of the acute infectious diseases. Their passage is largely by air, via droplets exhaled by carriers, or in the case of smallpox also by contact with the matter in the pustules that characterized the disease. Other deadly diseases were transmitted by intermediate vectors: Typhus, bubonic plague, yellow fever, and malaria were the most significant of these, and were transmitted by lice, fleas, and mosquitoes. Here a whole series of complex factors was brought into play before an epidemic stage was reached and the disease took permanent root in the Americas. It is not surprising, then, that measles, smallpox, and influenza were probably the first killer maladies in the New World, doing their damage for over half a century before typhus was introduced, to be followed by the plague, with yellow fever and cholera coming much later.

More than 90 percent of the Amerindians were killed by foreign infection. Based on travels in New Netherland, Adriaen Van der Donck observed in 1656 that "the Indians . . . affirm, that before the arrival of the Christians, and before the small pox broke out amongst them, they were ten times as numerous as they now are, and that their population had been melted down by this disease, whereof nine-tenths of them have died."[9] In spite of variations in mortality, the story was the same everywhere in the Americas. From the Caribbean to coastal Brazil, and northward to New England and New France, no group was spared, although highland peoples fared relatively better than those living along humid tropical coasts.

At the same time, many of the early European settlers in the New World suffered from poor health. The first colonial experiments faced initial "dying days" sometimes presenting weeks, even months of starvation, disease, and premature death. The eighteen men Columbus

9 Adriaen Van der Donck, A Description of the New Netherlands (New York: New York Historical Society, Collections, 2nd series, 1:125–242, 1841), p. 183, cited by Francis Jennings, The Invasion of America. Indians, Colonialism, and the Cant of Conquest (Chapel Hill: University of North Carolina Press, 1975), p. 24.

left behind on Hispaniola in January 1493 were dead by the time the second expedition across the Atlantic returned to the Caribbean. The record is shrouded, for the Arawaks at first were unwilling to disclose fully the reasons for the death of their unwelcome visitors, and given the small number of Europeans, it is likely that most were killed outright by the islanders rather than dying by starvation or disease. But the second expedition carried illness that afflicted Spaniards too. We have seen that many were laid low for several weeks, with extended and often halting recuperation. European susceptibilities were probably accentuated by new diets. The Spaniards were loath to try unknown foods, even if these might be more healthy than their own diets. Of the original 1,500 men of the second fleet of 1493, barely 200 survived in the Indies a quarter of a century later.

The killer epidemics for the Amerindians tended to come in waves, some exceptionally virulent, others more benign. The normal periodicity paralleled human generations, twenty-five to thirty years. Explosive outbursts of highly mortal epidemics took place only when there was a sufficient population density of susceptible individuals.[10] In Europe the acute infectious communicable diseases afflicted primarily children. In the New World adults were often affected too, with deadly consequences. Even the creoles tended to suffer higher mortality than the Europeans, for it took time for the Old World diseases to become endemic, infecting the young as they did normally in Europe. With the passage of time, the level of mortality for the Amerindian might be expected to decline. A lowering in the number of deaths from a particular disease would not be quick but would extend over a period of several generations. In the Americas, Old World disease mortality varied only slightly in the century and a half after contact, reaching similarly elevated mortality levels during the first four generations. Mortality of the mid-seventeenth century in many cases was just as high as it was at the time of the first encounter. Continuous exposure of a population to the smallpox virus might result in lower mortality after several generations, but 150 years is not a long enough time to make a significant difference. For the lower mortality levels, the disease would be endemic, so that almost continuously each generation would be exposed during childhood. But it took decades before the

10 Thomas M. Whitmore, *Disease and Death in Early Colonial Mexico. Simulating Amerindian Depopulation* (Boulder, CO: Westview Press, 1992), examines periodicity.

acute European diseases became endemic in the Americas. Indeed, many argue that smallpox never was endemic in America. Gelfand, for example, states that in New France it "never settled into the endemic childhood pattern characteristic of eighteenth-century French cities."[11] And tragically it was not one disease but wave after wave of new illnesses hitting in rapid succession that resulted in the most damage to native populations. The combination of smallpox, measles, typhus, malaria, typhoid, mumps, influenza, yellow fever, and, later, cholera, took a terrible toll of human lives.[12] The impact of two, three, or even four distinct diseases coinciding in a short period, as took place in Andean America in the late 1580s, was devastating. When such sicknesses coincided, the mortality levels were fearsome; 50, 60, 70 percent of those infected succumbed to the illnesses, for if they became infected while they were convalescing, they were usually too weak to withstand the second or third onslaught of alien disease.

The native response varied, but in no case was the reaction really effective. The first attempts to cure the sickness, using traditional medicine, were without success. Among some peoples, sweat baths followed by immersion in cold water killed people more frequently than it cured the infected. Furthermore, European medicine was equally ineffective, so the nature of the individual's experience with foreign infection was dependent to some degree on general health and nutrition. The Amerindian's response was also based on gender and age and on health care during the critical period of fever and convalescence. When the native populace fled in fear, as often happened, the victim was left to his or her own devices, and too frequently the weak died without food or water.

Throughout the Americas, flight was a common reaction of those who saw disaster coming. But attempting to evade the onslaught was usually not effective, for the sickness could be already incubating, only to break out in the unhappy victim dozens of kilometers from where the escape had been initiated. Bolting did little to protect in cases

---

11 Toby Gelfand, "Medicine in New France," in *Medicine in the New World. New Spain, New France, and New England*, ed. Ronald L. Numbers (Knoxville: University of Tennessee Press, 1987), p. 77.

12 Typhoid must have contributed heavily to disease-related deaths from the time it reached America. Indeed, it was likely the most significant killer of the first European settlers at Jamestown. Its symptoms are easy to confuse with typhus; in fact (personal communication from Kenneth Kiple) "the two [were] not disentangled until the middle of the 19th century."

where an intermediate vector was a reservoir of infection. Often an epidemic might appear to leapfrog from one spot to another, leaving some sectors relatively unscathed while other regions faced the full fury of the disease.

The natural flow of epidemics followed normal trade and communications routes between groups of people. Even the sea did not act as a barrier to the transfer of disease. Amerindian water-faring technology was advanced enough to permit voyages of hundreds of miles. Columbus and the first Europeans to enter the Caribbean were struck by the number of both small and large canoes with outriggers that plied the relatively calm waters of the inland sea. These craft transported ample numbers of people and all their artifacts, as well as their pests. Contact between the Greater and Lesser Antilles and the coast of mainland South America was constant, and regular relations existed with the Bahamas. On the east and west coasts of La Florida, small craft moved up and down the peninsula among the mangroves or behind barrier islands. Exchange was largely localized, but there was constant contact between ethnic groups at the peripheries of their territories. That contact was continuous enough to allow the free passage of pathogens. Pre-Columbian exchange existed along the Pacific coast of Andean America. Sailors associated with Francisco Pizarro's second expedition southward from Panama encountered large balsa rafts carrying dozens of persons, along with foodstuffs and trade goods. Furthermore, the tributaries of the Amazon basin acted as roads that permitted the constant movement of people. The mouths of the great river systems were touched by the Europeans relatively early in their reconnaissance of America, from the beginning of the sixteenth century as Amerigo Vespucci and Vicente Yáñez Pinzón entered the fresh waters of the Orinoco and Amazon, and Juan de Solís the Rio de la Plata in 1516. And by the early 1540s, Europeans actually moved downstream – the remnants of the Hernando de Soto expedition in the case of the Mississippi, and Francisco de Orellana coming from the headwaters of the Amazon. Thus, epidemics could be carried along the coasts of America and into the interior by major river systems, just as they might be transferred on foot in arid regions. There was no important natural barrier in the Americas, save the one that had perhaps screened the earliest waves of migrants from the Old World, the Arctic. Both mountain chains and deserts could be, and were, skirted by native migrants. Foreign disease, once introduced, extended as long as the chain of infection continued unbroken.

Religion provided another native response to disease-related death. Amerindians came quickly to associate the arrival of Europeans with sickness and excessive mortality. The mere arrival of the brown- and black-robed emissaries of a new religion seemed to cause death. One of the first things the Europeans did as they came into contact with the non-Christian peoples of America was to strip authority from the native priests and shamans because they were the guardians of the old demonistic lore. That group, or at least those who did not embrace the religion of the conquerors, held a deep-rooted antipathy toward the Christian deities. The native priests, steadfastly and often under cover of darkness and far from the eyes of the *doctrineros*, continued to appease the old religious forces and tried to sabotage the success of the Christian friars and their acolytes. The violent reaction of the Tupi-speaking shamans on Brazil's coast was no aberration. The messianic Santiadade movement of the 1560s centering on the Bahia district called for a return to the old order; the settlers would become food for the Tupi. As one Jesuit contemporary in the Portuguese colony bitterly complained, "The sorcerers delude them with a thousand follies and lies . . . preaching that we kill them with baptism, and proving this because many of them *do* die."[13]

At times some Amerindians attempted to use the power of disease to improve their own relative position. In New England, Squanto actually concocted a story that the English had hidden the plague "under the floor of their storehouse. . . . When Squanto hinted that he could influence the English to spring the killer from its lair, his stature rose to new heights, as did the Indians' fear of the colonists." The Puritans found out, and told the Indians that Squanto's claims were untrue; even they did not have that kind of power. The English went on to confide to the natives "that the God whom they served had Power to send that or any other Disease upon those that should doe any Wrong to his People."[14] The natives were probably unable to

---

13 John Hemming, *Red Gold: The Conquest of the Brazilian Indians* (Cambridge, MA: Harvard University Press, 1978), p. 141. B. J. Barickman, " 'Tame Indians,' 'Wild Heathens,' and Settlers in Southern Bahia in the Late Eighteenth and Early Nineteenth Centuries," *The Americas* 51(1995):330, points to violent reaction of the Aimoré backcountry non-Tupi in the 1570s when they came under pressure from coastal settlers. They attacked both the Portuguese and the surrounding Tupinikin, devastating the sugar economy.

14 Alden T. Vaughan, *New England Frontier. Puritans and Indians 1620–1675* (Boston: Little, Brown, 1965), p. 77.

make the distinction, and the fear of potential use of disease by the English probably helped keep the natives in check.

When the full disaster of conquest and subjugation under a colonial regime of forced or semiforced labor that had been wrought on them became evident, Amerindians tended to direct their fury toward Christian priests. The old forces were petitioned to bring back a better age and to throw off the yoke of the foreigners. The Taki Onkoy movement, which exploded in the 1560s in the central Andes, was just one of the nativist regeneration movements. The leaders of the group argued that the people had forsaken their traditional deities, and that only by a return to the veneration of the ancient *huacas* could the people be delivered. The extirpator of idolatries Cristóbal de Albornoz, who found and described the beliefs of the adherents of this "dancing sickness," or Taki Onkoy, reported that the natives believed that the spiritual forces of Pachacamac and Titicaca would join to throw out the foreigners. In addition, the Spaniards henceforth would be plagued by disease and death as the Andean Americans had been. Both Luis de Olvera, curate of the Cathedral of Cuzco, and Cristóbal Ximénez, of the Indian parish of Nuestra Señora de Belén of Cuzco, testified that Albornoz found that the natives believed

that the Spaniards of this land would come quickly to an end, because the huacas commanded diseases to descend and kill them all; they [the huacas] were angered with the Indians who became Christians, and if the Indians wanted sicknesses and deaths not to befall them, rather they have full health and an increase in their possessions, they should renounce the Christianity they had received, and stop using Christian names, nor eat nor dress in Castilian things.[15]

Thus the natives, through the return to their ancient huacas, would use the force of disease to turn the tables on their conquerors. America would be reconquered for Americans by disease!

The link between epidemic disease and ease of conquest, as in the retaking of the Aztec capital and the fratricidal strife in the Inca

15 Luis Millones, ed., *El retorno de las huacas: Estudios y documentos sobre el Taki Onqoy, Siglo XVI* (Lima: Instituto de Estudios Peruanos, 1990), pp. 178, 191; Sabine MacCormack, *Religion in the Andes. Vision and Imagination in Early Colonial Peru* (Princeton: Princeton University Press, 1991), pp. 181–204, provides important coverage of the movement and of the purification ritual of Citua, which also relates to sickness.

world after the death of Huayna Capac, was recognized by Spanish contemporaries. Disease was a powerful tool on the side of the Europeans who entered an alien land where they were outnumbered a thousand to one. Ulrich Schmidel honestly admitted that without the passage of an epidemic coinciding with the Europeans' onward march, exploration and subjugation of Paraguay would have been far different. A participant in the Hernando de Soto expedition of Florida expressed a similar sentiment. Had the Europeans knowingly used disease to kill native Americans, then clearly disease would have been a stronger and more reliable weapon than the sword. Furthermore, sickness often preceded the arrival of the newcomers and debilitated the natives before the Europeans ever met them face to face. The devastation caused by illness was the most tragic of all the consequences of the discovery of the Americas. Whether the infection was carried back to the Old World by those returning to their homelands or transported to the Americas aboard the ships and within the bodies of the newcomers, the impact was the same: infection, illness, debilitation, and painful and untimely death. Acute communicable diseases opened the way for European domination of the unfortunates vanquished through the epidemiological exchange.

Yet the rapid demise of the Amerindian population under Spanish rule did not please the newcomers, who had expected to use native labor on their estates and in their mines. The demographic disaster that hit the Caribbean in the first half century was bemoaned not only by Las Casas but by a wide group of clergy, bureaucrats, and settlers. The disappearance of the Taino led quickly to the importation of increasing numbers of African workers, taken as slaves and transported across the Atlantic under horrendous conditions. But where native populations were dense, and less affected by epidemic death than in tropical and subtropical lowlands, the Spaniards attempted to stem the tide of demographic collapse. The Indian ordinances of Viceroy Francisco de Toledo in the viceroyalty of Peru in the 1570s required that there be a physician in each large Indian town. Quarantine was used by the Spanish in the Andes in the late 1580s to stop the progression of mortal epidemics coming from the Gulf port cities of what later became Colombia. Regulations to check the abuses of holders of Indian grants, the *encomenderos*, were enacted for both Christian and medical reasons. The Spanish, at least from the time of the New Laws of the 1540s, attempted to stop the most flagrant abuse of native Americans under their control. One practical reason was to prevent their extinction so that they could provide labor.

Each European nation in America had its own idea of who the Indians were and what role they were to play in colonial society. The European view was not static; it changed over time. The first Spaniards to enter the circum-Caribbean were far less concerned with the Amerindian's welfare than those who came a half century later. The English, especially those who settled in New England, saw the native American as standing in the way of their erection of "God's City on a Hill." Even elsewhere in the English colonies established along the Atlantic seaboard of North America in the generation following Jamestown in 1607, the Indians were seen as savages who lived in the wrong place and were to be removed in any way that might be necessary. In the early seventeenth century, some of the first settlers of New England rejoiced that so many natives had died that the land seemed to be opened to them by Divine Providence. John Winthrop, for example, defended the Massachusetts venture, writing that "God hath consumed the natives with such a great plague in these parts, so as there be few inhabitants left."[16] A few years later, William Wood, referring to the smallpox epidemic of 1633, said that Indian losses had been brought on by the quarrelsome nature of the Indians and by God's desire to "make room for the following part of his army." But the early Puritans did not mention that they took direct action to assist and speed up "Divine" intervention. The eighteenth and nineteenth centuries, however, provided concrete examples of germ warfare, in which blankets infected with the smallpox virus were given by Anglo settlers to the Indians.

There are occasional documentary glimpses of that unsavory reality. In 1763 correspondence between Sir Jeffrey Amherst, commander of British forces in North America, and Colonel Henry Bouquet, in charge of the Ohio frontier, Amherst suggested that smallpox might be introduced among native-American populations. He wrote, "Could it not be contrived to send the Small Pox among those disaffected tribes of Indians? We must on this occasion use every stratagem [sic] in our power to reduce them." Bouquet responded, "I will try to innoculate [them] with some blankets that might fall into their hands." Colonel Bouquet continued, in a style appropriate to an adherent of the Black Legend, "I wish we could make use of the

---

16 Robert C. Winthrop, *Life and Letters of John Winthrop*, 2 vols. (Boston: Ticknor & Fields, 1864–67), 1:312.

Spanish method, to hunt them with English dogs, supported by rangers and some light horse, who would, I think, effectively extirpate or remove that vermin." Amherst responded, "You will do well to try to innoculate the Indians by means of blankets as well as to try every other method that can serve to extirpate this execrable race." Amherst also said he would be "glad if your scheme for hunting them down by dogs could take effect, but England is at too great a distance to think of that at present." Captain Simeon Ecuyler of the Royal Americans recorded in his journal that "out of our regard for them [two Indian chiefs] we gave them two blankets and a handkerchief out of the smallpox hospital. I hope it will have the desired effect." Furthermore, it is recorded that the firm of Levy, Trent and Company charged the Crown in June 1763 for "sundries got to replace in kind those which were taken from the people in the Hospital to Convey the Small-pox to the Indians viz: 2 Blankets at 20/1 OO, 1 Silk Handkerchief LO/ O & Linens do 3/6." Subsequent documents indicate that several knew of the project; even General Thomas Gage endorsed it.[17]

Far to the south, on the Chilean frontier, it would be smallpox, in a devastating epidemic of the early 1790s, that would for a time break, some believe, the resistance of the fiercely independent Mapuche and bring about their halting integration into colonial society.[18] In the twentieth century, the conquest of Amerindian America by disease continues, as Brazilian settlers and miners transport infections intentionally to the native groups whose lands they covet.

No evidence has been encountered that the Spanish ever deliberately attempted to infect the Amerindians in the colonial era, perhaps because after the sixteenth century the native population had fallen to a low level in the core centers of settlement, the basin of Mexico, and the Andean heartland. In fact, by the time that approximately nine of ten native Americans had died, the Spanish tried hard to

17 The most complete description of Parkman's discovery of "germ warfare" more than a century previously is provided by Wilbur R. Jacobs, *Francis Parkman, Historian as Hero* (Austin: University of Texas Press, 1991), pp. 84–86, 199–200. Accounts provided by Russell Thornton, *American Indian Holocaust and Survival: A Population History since 1492* (Norman: University of Oklahoma Press, 1987), pp. 78–79, and by E. Wagner Stearn and Allen E. Stearn, *The Effect of Smallpox on the Destiny of the Amerindian* (Boston: Bruce Humphries, 1945), pp. 44–45, are misleading.

18 Fernando Casanueva, "Smallpox and War in Southern Chile in the Late Eighteenth Century," in *The Secret Judgments of God: Native Peoples and Old World Disease in Colonial Spanish America* (Norman: University of Oklahoma Press, 1992), ed. Noble David Cook and W. George Lovell, pp. 183–212.

preserve and even augment remaining populations. By the end of the first century after uniting the disease pools of the Old and New Worlds, the Spanish realized that they had to try to protect those Amerindians who had survived, because a large and healthy native-American labor force was critical for maintenance of the colonial regimes and the prosperity of the Iberian homeland. Alchon described public-health measures employed in the Audiencia of Quito that included quarantine and the burning of infected household goods.[19] The same was done farther south, in the Lima and Cuzco districts, under careful supervision by the Viceroy Conde de Villar, who had used similar techniques to block entrance of the bubonic plague into Seville, where he had been chief administrator in the early 1580s. Quarantine may have been used in Boston in 1647, when ships arrived from the West Indies. Local quarantine may have been attempted in the English settlement of East Hampton, on Long Island, in 1662, to prevent smallpox that had infected local Indians from assaulting townsmen. New York may have first used the practice in 1690, when a shipload of smallpox-infected slaves came from the island of St. Nevis.[20]

Time after time in Mesoamerica, the authors of the Mayan texts poignantly lamented the loss of an earlier world. The text of the Chilam Balam de Chumayel, though not in final form until 1782, eloquently expresses the feelings of the peoples of the Yucatán, their belief that before the arrival of the Europeans their world had been a better, more orderly, and healthier place: "Then all was well. There was in them wisdom. There was then no sin. There was holy devotion in them." The authors of this account stated that the transfer of Christianity to Mesoamerica did not bring greater knowledge. Neither did the clerics create a less sin-filled existence in Mesoamerica. Instead, after time they came to believe that before the arrival of the bearded white men from across the sea, "Healthfully they lived. There was not then illness; no aching bones; no fever among them; no smallpox, there were no burning chests, there was not pain in the belly, no consumption. Their bodies were upright then."[21] Theirs was a vision of a lost paradise, a view that combined neatly with the

19 Suzanne Austin Alchon, Native Society and Disease in Colonial Ecuador (Cambridge: Cambridge University Press, 1991), pp. 41–42.
20 Donald R. Hopkins, Princes and Peasants: Smallpox in History (Chicago: University of Chicago Press, 1983), pp. 238–39.
21 Miguel Rivera, ed., Chilam Balam de Chumayel (Madrid: Historia 16, 1986) p. 72.

Christian belief system, with its emphasis on a strong messianic figure and a paradise that would come. For centuries the plaint of Mayan peoples was voiced without response. The haunting chant of the era of conquest and premature death continued to the end of the colonial regime: "The mortality was terrible. Your grandfathers died, and with them died the son of the king and his brothers and kinsmen. So it was that we became orphans, Oh my sons! So we became when we were young. All of us were thus. We were born to die!"

BIBLIOGRAPHY

Alchon, Suzanne Austin. "Disease, Population and Public Health in Eighteenth-Century Quito." In *The Secret Judgments of God: Native Peoples and Old World Disease in Colonial Spanish America,* ed. Noble David Cook and W. George Lovell, pp. 159–82. Norman: University of Oklahoma Press, 1992.

Alchon, Suzanne Austin. *Native Society and Disease in Colonial Ecuador.* Cambridge: Cambridge University Press, 1991.

Alden, Dauril, and Joseph C. Miller. "Out of Africa. The Slave Trade and the Transmission of Smallpox to Brazil, 1560–1831." *Journal of Interdisciplinary History* 18(1987):195–224.

Alden, Dauril, and Joseph C. Miller. "Unwanted Cargoes: The Origin and Dissemination of Smallpox via the Slave Trade, c. 1560–1830." In *The African Exchange: Toward a Biological History of Black People,* ed. Kenneth F. Kiple, pp. 35–109. Durham: Duke University Press, 1987.

Alexander, Michael, ed. *Discovering the New World.* New York: Harper & Row, 1976.

Altman, Ida. *Emigrants and Society: Extremadura and America in the Sixteenth Century.* Berkeley: University of California Press, 1989.

Amiama, Manuel A. "La población de Santo Domingo." *Clio* 115(1959):116–34.

Anales de Tecamachalco. "Crónica local y colonial en idioma nahuatl, 1398 y 1590." In *Colección de documentos para la historia mexicana,* ed. Antonio Peñafiel. 6 vols. México: Secretaria de Fomento, 1897–1903.

Anderson, Gaylord West, and Margaret G. Arnstein. *Communicable Disease Control.* New York: Macmillan, 1956.

Archila, Ricardo. *Historia de la medicina en Venezuela: Epoca colonial.* Caracas: Tipografía Vargas, 1961.

Arcos, Gualberto. *Evolución de la medicina en el Ecuador.* Quito: Casa de la Cultura Ecuatoriana, 1979.

Arcos, Gualberto. *La medicina en el Ecuador.* Quito: Tipográfico L. I. Fernández, 1933.

Ashburn, Percy M. *The Ranks of Death: A Medical History of the Conquest of America.* New York: Coward-McCann, 1947.

Assadourian, Carlos Sempat. "La crísis demográfica del siglo XVI y la transición del Tawantinsuyu al sistema mercantil colonial." In *Población y mano de obra en América Latina,* ed. Nicolás Sánchez-Albornoz, pp. 69–93. Madrid: Alianza Editorial, 1985.

Astrain, Antonio. *Historia de la compañía de Jesús en la asistencia de España.* Madrid: Administración de Razón y Fé, 1913.

Asturias, Francisco. *Historia de la medicina en Guatemala.* Guatemala: Editorial Universitaria, 1958.

Aten, Lawrence E. *Indians of the Upper Texas Coast.* New York: Academic Press, 1983.

Axtell, James. *Beyond 1492: Encounters in Colonial North America.* New York: Oxford University Press, 1992.

Axtell, James. *The Invasion Within. The Contest of Cultures in Colonial North America.* New York: Oxford University Press, 1985.

Bailes, Kendall E., ed. *Environmental History: Critical Issues in Comparative Perspective.* New York: University Press of America, 1985.

Bailey, Alfred G. *The Conflict of European and Eastern Algonkian Cultures, 1504–1700. A Study in Canadian Civilization.* Toronto: University of Toronto Press, 1969.

Baker, Brenda J., and George J. Armelagos. "The Origin and Antiquity of Syphilis: Paleopathological Diagnosis and Interpretation." *Current Anthropology* 29(1988):703–37.

Balcazar, Juan Manuel. *Historia de la medicina en Bolivia.* La Paz: Ediciones Juventud, 1956.

Ball, A. P. "Measles." In *A World Geography of Human Diseases,* ed. G. Melvyn Howe, pp. 237–54. New York: Academic Press, 1977.

Ballesteros Rodríguez, Juan. *La peste en Córdoba.* Córdoba: Diputación Provincial, 1982.

Barickman, B. J. " 'Tame Indians,' 'Wild Heathens,' and Settlers in Southern Bahia in the Late Eighteenth and Early Nineteenth Centuries." *The Americas* 51(1995):325–68.

Barrow, Mark V., Jerry D. Niswander, and Robert Fortune. *Health and Disease of American Indians North of Mexico: A Bibliography, 1810–1969.* Gainesville: University of Florida Press, 1972.

Benenson, Abram S., ed. *Control of Communicable Diseases in Man.* 13th ed. Washington, DC: American Public Health Association, 1981.

Benzoni, Girolamo. *Historia del nuevo mundo.* Madrid: Alianza Editorial, 1989. Originally published in 1572.

Bernáldez, Andrés. *Memorias del reinado de los Reyes Católicos.* Madrid, 1962.

Berte, J. P. "Les epidemies au Mexique au XVIe siècle." *Asclepio* 35(1983):357–63.

Bertonio, Ludovico. *Vocabulario de la lengua aymara* (1612 facs. ed.). Cochabamba: CERES, 1984.

Betanzos, Juan de. *Suma y narración de los Incas.* Madrid: Atlas, 1987.

Bett, Walter R. *The History and Conquest of Common Diseases.* Norman: University of Oklahoma Press, 1954.

Biggar, H. P., ed. *The Voyages of Jacques Cartier.* Ottawa: F. A. Acland, 1924.

Black, Francis L. "Infectious Diseases in Primitive Societies." *Science* 187 (1975):515–18.

Black, Francis L., Francisco de P. Pinheiro, Walter J. Hier, and Richard V. Lee. "Epidemiology of Infectious Disease: The Example of Measles." In *Health and Disease in Tribal Societies,* pp. 115–35. Ciba Foundation Symposium 49. Amsterdam: Elsevier, 1976.

Borah, Woodrow. "America as Model: The Demographic Impact of European Expansion upon the Non-European World." *Actas y memorias del XXXV Congreso Internacional de Americanistas.* México, 3(1964): 379–87.

Borah, Woodrow. "Introduction." In *The Secret Judgments of God: Native Peoples and Old World Disease in Colonial Spanish America,* ed. Noble David Cook and W. George Lovell, pp. 3–19. Norman: University of Oklahoma Press, 1992.

Borah, Woodrow, and Sherburne F. Cook. *Essays in Population History.* 3 vols. Berkeley: University of California Press, 1971–79.

Borrego Plá, María del Carmen. *Cartagena de Indias en el siglo XVI.* Seville: Escuela de Estudios Hispano-americanos, 1983.

Bouysse Cassagne, Thérèse. *La identidad aymara. Aproximación histórica (Siglo XV, Siglo XVI).* La Paz: HISBOL, 1987.

Boxer, Charles R. *Two Pioneers of Tropical Medicine: Garcia d'Orta and Nicolas Monardes.* London: Hispanic and Luso-Brazilian Councils, 1963.

Bradford, William. *Of Plymouth Plantation.* New York: Modern Library, 1967.

Brading, David A. *The First America: The Spanish Monarchy, Creole Patriots, and the Liberal State 1492–1867.* Cambridge: Cambridge University Press, 1991.

Brau, Salvador. *La colonización del Puerto Rico.* San Juan: Instituto de Cultura Puertorriqueña, 1969.

Brinton, Daniel G., ed. *The Annals of the Cakchiquels.* Philadelphia: Library of Aboriginal American Literature, 1885.

Brooks, Francis J. "Revising the Conquest of Mexico: Smallpox, Sources and Populations." *Journal of Interdisciplinary History* 24(1993):1–29.

Brothwell, Don R. "Yaws." In *The Cambridge World History of Human Disease,* ed. Kenneth F. Kiple, pp. 1096–1100. Cambridge: Cambridge University Press, 1993.

Browne, Suzanne Austin. "The Effects of Epidemic Disease in Colonial Ecuador." Ph.D. diss. Durham: Duke University, 1984.

Burnet, MacFarlane. *Natural History of Infectious Disease*. Cambridge: Cambridge University Press, 1953.

Bustamante, Miguel E. *La fiebre amarilla en México y su origen en América*. México, 1958.

Busto Duthurburu, José Antonio del. *Historia general del Perú, descubrimiento y conquista*. Lima: Studium, 1978.

Cabello de Balboa, Miguel. *Miscelánea antártica*. Lima: San Marcos, 1951.

Calero, Luis F. *Chiefdoms under Siege: Spain's Rule and Native Adaptation in the Southern Colombian Andes, 1535–1700*. Albuquerque: University of New Mexico Press, 1997.

Calvete de Estrella, Juan Cristóbal. *Rebelión de Pizarro en el Perú y vida de don Pedro Gasca. Crónicas del Perú*. Madrid: Biblioteca de Autores Españoles, 1964.

Carmichael, Ann G., and Silverstein, Arthur M. "Smallpox in Europe before the Seventeenth Century: Virulent Killer or Benign Disease?" *Journal of the History of Medicine and Allied Sciences* 42(1987):147–68.

Carmona García, Juan I. *El sistema de la hospitalidad pública en la Sevilla del antiguo régimen*. Seville: Diputación Provincial, 1979.

Carreras Panchon, Antonio. *La peste y los médicos en la España del renacimiento*. Salamanca: Universidad de Salamanca, 1976.

Casanueva, Fernando. "Smallpox and War in Southern Chile in the Late Eighteenth Century." In *The Secret Judgments of God: Native Peoples and Old World Disease in Colonial Spanish America*, ed. Noble David Cook and W. George Lovell, pp. 185–214. Norman: University of Oklahoma Press, 1992.

Chandler, David L. *Health and Slavery in Colonial Colombia*. New York: Arno Press, 1981.

Chaunu, Pierre, and Huguette Chaunu. *Seville et l'Atlantique (1504–1650)*. 12 vols. Paris: Colin, 1956–60.

Chiappelli, Fredi, ed. *First Images of America: The Impact of the New World on the Old*. 2 vols. Berkeley: University of California Press, 1978.

Chimalpahin, Domingo Francisco de San Antón Muñón. "Die Relationen Chimalpahins zur Geschichte Mexicos." *Teil 2: Das Jahrhundert nach der Conquista*. Hamburg: Cram de Gruyter, 1965.

Christie, A. B. "Smallpox." In *A World Geography of Diseases*, ed. G. M. Howe, pp. 255–70. New York: Academic Press, 1977.

Cieza de León, Pedro de. *Crónica del Perú: Primera parte*. Lima: Pontificia Universidad Católica del Perú, 1984.

Cieza de León, Pedro de. *Obras completas*. 3 vols. Madrid: Consejo Superior de Investigaciones Científicas, 1984–85.

Cieza de León, Pedro de. *Señorio de los Incas.* Lima: Pontificia Universidad Católica del Perú, 1984.

Cipolla, Carlo M. *Christofano and the Plague: A Study in the History of Public Health in the Age of Galileo.* Berkeley: University of California Press, 1973.

Cobo, Bernabé. *Historia del nuevo mundo.* 2 vols. Madrid: Real Academia de la Historia, 1956.

Cohen, J. M., ed. *The Four Voyages of Christopher Columbus.* Baltimore: Penguin Books, 1969.

Colmenares, Germán. *Encomienda y población en la provincia de Pamplona (1549–1650).* Bogotá: Universidad de los Andes, 1969.

Columbus, Christopher. *The Log of Christopher Columbus,* trans. Robert H. Fuson. Camden, ME: International Marine Publishing, 1987.

Cook, Noble David. *Demographic Collapse: Indian Peru, 1520–1620.* Cambridge: Cambridge University Press, 1981.

Cook, Noble David. "Disease and Depopulation of Hispaniola, 1492–1518." *Colonial Latin American Review* 2(1993):213–45.

Cook, Noble David. *People of the Colca Valley: A Population Study.* Boulder, CO: Westview Press, 1982.

Cook, Noble David. "La población de la parroquia de Yanahuara, 1738–47." In *Collaguas I,* ed. Franklin Pease G. Y., pp. 13–34. Lima: Pontificia Universidad Católica del Perú, 1977.

Cook, Noble David, and W. George Lovell, eds. *The Secret Judgments of God: Native Peoples and Old World Disease in Colonial Spanish America.* Norman: University of Oklahoma Press, 1992.

Cook, Noble David, and W. George Lovell. "Unraveling the Web of Disease." In *The Secret Judgments of God: Native Peoples and Old World Disease in Colonial Spanish America,* ed. Noble David Cook and W. George Lovell, pp. 215–44. Norman: University of Oklahoma Press, 1992.

Cook, Noble David, and José Hernández Palomo. "Epidemias en Triana (Sevilla, 1660–1865)." *Annali della facolta di Economia e Commercio della Universita di Bari* 31(1992):53–81.

Cook, Sherburne F. "Significance of Disease in the Extinction of the New England Indian." *Human Biology* 45(1973):485–508.

Cooper, Donald B. *Epidemic Disease in Mexico City, 1761–1813: An Administrative, Social, and Medical Study.* Austin: University of Texas Press, 1965.

Cooper, Donald B. "The New 'Black Death': Cholera in Brazil, 1855–1856." In *The African Exchange. Toward a Biological History of Black People,* ed. Kenneth F. Kiple, pp. 235–56. Durham: Duke University Press, 1987.

Cooper, Donald B., and Kenneth F. Kiple. "Yellow Fever." In *The Cambridge World History of Human Disease,* ed. Kenneth F. Kiple, pp. 1100–1107. Cambridge: Cambridge University Press, 1993.

Córdova, Efrén. "La encomienda y la desaparación de los indios en las Antillas mayores." *Caribbean Studies* 8(1968):23–49.

Cortés, Hernando. *Cartas de relación*. México: Editorial Porrúa, 1971.

Covarrubias Orozco, Sebastián de. *Tesoro de la lengua castellana o española*. Madrid: Editorial Castalia, 1994.

Crosby, Alfred W. "Conquistador y Pestilencia: The First New World Pandemic and the Fall of the Great Indian Empires." *Hispanic American Historical Review* 47(1967):321–37.

Crosby, Alfred W. *Ecological Imperialism: The Biological Expansion of Europe, 900–1900*. Cambridge: Cambridge University Press, 1986.

Crosby, Alfred W. *Epidemic and Peace, 1918*. Westport, CT: Greenwood Press, 1976.

Crosby, Alfred W. *The Columbian Exchange: Biological and Cultural Consequences of 1492*. Westport, CT: Greenwood Press, 1972.

Crosby, Alfred W. "Virgin Soil Epidemics as a Factor in the Aboriginal Depopulation in America." *William and Mary Quarterly* 33(1976): 289–99.

Curtin, Philip D. *Death by Migration: Europe's Encounter with the Tropical World in the Nineteenth Century*. Cambridge: Cambridge University Press, 1989.

Curtin, Philip D. "Epidemiology and the Slave Trade." *Political Science Quarterly* 83(1968):190–216.

Davies, Hunter. *In Search of Columbus*. London: Sinclair-Stevenson, 1991.

Dean, Warren. "Indigenous Populations of the São Paulo–Rio de Janeiro Coast: Trade, Aldeamento, Slavery and Extinction." *Revista Histórica* (São Paulo) 117(1984):3–26.

Dean, Warren. "Las poblaciones indígenas del litoral brasileño de São Paulo a Rio de Janeiro: Comercio, esclavitud, reducción y extinción." In *Población y mano de obra en América Latina*, ed. Nicolás Sánchez-Albornoz, pp. 25–52. Madrid: Alianza América, 1985.

Denevan, William M., ed. *The Native Population of the Americas in 1492*. 2nd ed. Madison: University of Wisconsin Press, 1992.

Denevan, William M. "The Pristine Myth: The Landscape of the Americas in 1492." *Annals of the Association of American Geographers* 82(1992): 369–85.

Dibble, Charles E. *Codex en Cruz*. 2 vols. Salt Lake City: University of Utah Press, 1981.

Dixon, C. W. *Smallpox*. London: J. and A. Churchill, 1962.

Dobyns, Henry F. "An Outline of Andean Epidemic History to 1720." *Bulletin of the History of Medicine* 37(1963):493–515.

Dobyns, Henry F. "Disease Transfer at Contact." *Annual Review of Anthropology* 22(1993):273–91.

Dobyns, Henry F. "Estimating Aboriginal Populations: An Appraisal of Techniques with a New Hemispheric Estimate." *Current Anthropology* 7(1966):395–449.

Dobyns, Henry F. *Their Number Become Thinned: Native American Population Dynamics in Eastern North America.* Knoxville: University of Tennessee Press, 1983.

Duffy, John. *Epidemics in Colonial America.* Baton Rouge: Louisiana State University Press, 1953.

Duffy, John. "Smallpox and the Indians in the American Colonies." *Bulletin of the History of Medicine* 25(1951):324–41.

Dunn, Frederick L. "Malaria." In *The Cambridge World History of Human Disease*, ed. Kenneth F. Kiple, pp. 855–62. Cambridge: Cambridge University Press, 1993.

Esteve Barba, Francisco. *Historiografía indiana.* Madrid: Editorial Gredos, 1964.

Evans, Brian. "Death in Aymaya of Upper Peru." In *The Secret Judgments of God: Native Peoples and Old World Disease in Colonial Spanish America*, ed. Noble David Cook and W. George Lovell, pp. 144–60. Norman: University of Oklahoma Press, 1992.

Federmann, Nikolaus. *Historia indiana.* Trans. Juan Friede. Madrid: Artes Gráficas, 1958.

Fernández-Armesto, Felipe. *Columbus.* New York: Oxford University Press, 1991.

Figueroa, Francisco de. *Relación de las misiones de la Compañía de Jesús en el país de los Maynas.* Madrid, 1904.

Figueroa Marroquin, Horacio. *Enfermedades de los conquistadores.* Guatemala: Universidad de San Carlos de Guatemala, 1983.

Fish, Suzanne, and Paul Fish. "Historic Demography and Ethnographic Analogy." *Early Georgia* 7(1979):29–43.

Fisher, F. J. "Influenza and Inflation in Tudor England." *Economic History Review* 18(1965):120–29.

Flinn, Michael W. *The European Demographic System, 1500–1820.* Baltimore: Johns Hopkins University Press, 1981.

Florescano, Enrique, and Elsa Malvido, eds. *Ensayos sobre la historia de las epidemias en México.* 2 vols. México: Instituto Mexicano del Seguro Social, 1980.

Floyd, T. S. *The Columbus Dynasty in the Caribbean, 1492 to 1526.* Albuquerque: University of New Mexico Press, 1973.

Franco, Francisco. *Libro de enfermedades contagiosas y de la preservación dellas.* Seville, 1569.

Friede, Juan. "Demographic Changes in the Mining Community of Muzo after the Plague of 1629." *Hispanic American Historical Review* 47(1967): 338–59.

Friede, Juan, ed. *Documentos inéditos para la historia de Colombia*. 10 vols. Bogotá: Academia Colombiana de Historia, 1955–60.

Friede, Juan. *Los quimbayas bajo la dominación española: Estudio documental (1539–1810)*. Bogotá: Banco de la República, 1963.

Fuentes y Guzmán, Francisco Antonio de. *Recordación Florida*. 3 vols. Guatemala: Sociedad de Geografía e Historia, 1932–33.

Gade, Daniel W. "Inca and Colonial Settlements, Coca Cultivation and Endemic Disease in the Tropical Forest." *Journal of Historical Geography* 5(1979):263–79.

Gage, Thomas. *The English American: A New Survey of the West Indies*. London: Routledge, 1928.

Gannon, Michael V. *The Cross in the Sand: The Early Catholic Church in Florida, 1513–1870*. Gainesville: University of Florida Press, 1965.

Ganson, Barbara J. "The Evueví of Paraguay: Adaptive Strategies and Responses to Colonialism, 1528–1811." *The Americas* 45(1989):461–88.

Gelfand, Toby. "Medicine in New France." In *Medicine in the New World: New Spain, New France, and New England*, ed. Ronald L. Numbers, pp. 64–100. Knoxville: University of Tennessee Press, 1987.

Gerhard, Peter. *A Guide to the Historical Geography of New Spain*. Rev. ed. Norman: University of Oklahoma Press, 1993.

Gibson, Charles. *The Aztecs under Spanish Rule: A History of the Indians of the Valley of Mexico, 1519–1810*. Stanford: Stanford University Press, 1964.

Gibson, Charles, ed. *The Black Legend: Anti-Spanish Attitudes in the Old World and in the New*. New York: Alfred A. Knopf, 1971.

Gil, Juan, and Consuelo Varela, eds. *Cartas de particulares a Colón y relaciones coetáneas*. Madrid: Alianza, 1984.

Gil, Juan, and Consuelo Varela, eds. *Temas colombinas*. Seville: 1986.

Grmek, Mirko D. *Diseases in the Ancient Greek World*. Baltimore: Johns Hopkins University Press, 1989.

Guerra, Francisco. "El efecto demográfico de las epidemias tras el descubrimiento de América." *Revista de Indias* 46(1986):41–58.

Guerra, Francisco. *Historia de la Medicina*. 2 vols. Madrid: Ediciones Norma, 1982.

Guerra, Francisco. "La epidemia americana de influenza en 1493." *Revista de Indias* 45(1985):325–47.

Guerra, Francisco. "The Dispute over Syphilis: Europe versus America." *Clio Medica* (Netherlands) 13(1978):39–62.

Guerra, Francisco. "The Earliest American Epidemic: The Influenza of 1493." *Social Science History* 12(1988):305–25.

Guerra, Francisco. "The Influence of Disease on Race, Logistics, and Colonization in the Antilles." *Journal of Tropical Medicine* 49 (1966):23–35.

Guerra, Francisco. "The Problem of Syphilis." In *First Images of America: The Impact of the New World on the Old*, ed. Fredi Chiappelli, pp. 845–51. 2 vols. Berkeley: University of California Press, 1975.

Guerra y Sánchez, Ramiro. *Historia de la nación cubana*. 10 vols. Havana: Editorial Historia de la Nación Cubana, 1952.

Hampe Martínez, Teodoro. *Don Pedro de la Gasca: su obra política en España y América*. Lima: Universidad Católica del Perú, 1989.

Hanke, Lewis. *The Spanish Struggle for Justice in the Conquest of America*. Boston: Little, Brown, 1965.

Haubrich, William S. *Medical Meanings: A Glossary of Word Origins*. New York: Harcourt Brace Jovanovich, 1984.

Hemming, John. *Red Gold: The Conquest of the Brazilian Indians*. Cambridge, MA: Harvard University Press, 1978.

Hemming, John. *The Conquest of the Incas*. London: Sphere Books, 1972.

Henige, David. "Counting the Encounter: The Pernicious Appeal of Verisimilitude." *Colonial Latin American Historical Review* 3(1993):325–61.

Henige, David. "On the Contact Population of Hispaniola: History as Higher Mathematics." *Hispanic American Historical Review* 58(1978):217–37.

Henige, David. "When Did Smallpox Reach the New World (and Why Does It Matter?)" In *Africans in Bondage: Studies in Slavery and the Slave Trade*, ed. Paul E. Lovejoy, pp. 11–26. Madison: University of Wisconsin Press, 1986.

Herrera y Tordesillas, Antonio de. *Historia general de los hechos de los castellanos en las islas y tierra firme del Mar Océano*. 17 vols. Madrid: Real Academia de la Historia, 1934.

Hoeppli, Rudolph. *Parasitic Diseases in Africa and the Western Hemisphere: Early Documentation and Transmission by the Slave Trade*. Basel, 1969.

Hoffman, Paul E. *A New Andalucia and a Way to the Orient: The American Southeast during the Sixteenth Century*. Baton Rouge: Louisiana State University Press, 1990.

Hopkins, Donald R. *Princes and Peasants: Smallpox in History*. Chicago: University of Chicago Press, 1983.

Humboldt, Alexander Freiherr von. *Ensayo político sobre el reino de la Nueva España*. México: Editorial Porrúa, 1966.

Jackson, Robert H. *Indian Population Decline. The Missions of Northwestern New Spain, 1687–1840*. Albuquerque: University of New Mexico Press, 1994.

Jacobs, Wilbur R. *Francis Parkman, Historian as Hero*. Austin: University of Texas Press, 1991.

Jarcho, Saul. "Jaundice during the Second Voyage of Columbus." *Revista de la Asociación de Salud Pública de Puerto Rico* 2(1958):24–27.

Jennings, Francis. *The Invasion of America: Indians, Colonialism, and the Cant of Conquest*. Chapel Hill: University of North Carolina Press, 1975.

Jiménez de la Espada, Marcos, ed. *Relaciones geográficas de Indias. Perú.* 3 vols. Madrid: Atlas, 1965.

Joralemon, Donald. "New World Depopulation and the Case of Disease." *Journal of Anthropological Research* 38(1982):108–27.

Karlen, Arno. *Man and Microbes: Disease and Plagues in History and Modern Times.* New York: G. P. Putnam's Sons, 1995.

Kiple, Kenneth F., ed. *The African Exchange: Toward a Biological History of Black People.* Durham: Duke University Press, 1987.

Kiple, Kenneth F., ed. *The Cambridge World History of Human Disease.* Cambridge: Cambridge University Press, 1993.

Kiple, Kenneth F. *The Caribbean Slave: A Biological History.* Cambridge: Cambridge University Press, 1984.

Klüpfel, Karl, ed. *N. Federmanns und H. Stadens Reisen in Südamerica 1529 bis 1555.* Stuttgart: Literarischer Verein, 1859.

Kramer, Wendy. *Encomienda Politics in Early Colonial Guatemala, 1524–1544.* Boulder, CO: Westview Press, 1994.

Krech, Shepard. "Disease, Starvation, and North Athapaskan Social Organization." *American Ethnologist* 5(1978):710–32.

Kroemer, Gunter. *Cuxiuara, o purus dos indigenas.* São Paulo: Ediciones Loyola, 1985.

Lamb, Ursula. *Frey Nicolás de Ovando: Gobernador de Indias, 1501–1509.* Madrid, 1956.

Landa, Diego de. *Yucatán before and after the Conquest.* New York: Dover, 1978.

Las Casas, Bartolomé de. *Historia de las Indias.* 3 vols. México: Fondo de Cultura Económica, 1951.

Las Casas, Bartolomé de. *Obras escogidas de fray Bartolomé de las Casas,* ed. Juan Pérez de Tudela, 5 vols. Madrid: Biblioteca de Autores Españoles, 1957–58.

Lastres, Juan B. *Historia de la medicina peruana.* 3 vols. Lima: San Marcos, 1951.

León-Portilla, Miguel, ed. *Broken Spears: The Aztec Account of the Conquest of Mexico.* Boston: Beacon Press, 1992.

Leroy y Cassa, Jorge. *La primera epidemia de fiebre amarilla en la Habana, en 1649.* Havana, 1930.

Léry, Jean de. *History of a Voyage to the Land of Brazil Otherwise Called America.* Berkeley: University of California Press, 1993.

Levillier, Roberto, ed. *Gobernantes del Perú: Cartas y papeles siglo XVI.* 14 vols. Madrid: Sucesores de Rivadeneyra, 1925.

Lipschutz, Alejandro. "La despoblación de los indios después de la conquista." *América Indígena* 26(1966):229–47.

Lizárraga, Reginaldo de. *Descripción breve de toda la tierra de Perú, Tucumán, Rio de la Plata y Chile.* Madrid: Atlas, 1968.

Lizárraga, Reginaldo de. *Descripción de las Indias*. Lima: Pequeños Grandes Libros de Historia Americana, 1946.

Lockhart, James. *Men of Cajamarca: A Social and Biographical Study of the First Conquerors of Peru*. Austin: University of Texas Press, 1972.

Lockhart, James. *Spanish Peru, 1532–1560: A Colonial Society*. Madison: University of Wisconsin Press, 1968.

Lockhart, James. *We People Here: Nahuatl Accounts of the Conquest of Mexico*. Berkeley: University of California Press, 1993.

López Austin, Alfredo. *Textos de medicina nahuatl*. México: UNAM, 1975.

López Austin, Alfredo. *The Human Body and Ideology: Concepts of the Ancient Nahuas*. 2 vols. Salt Lake City: University of Utah Press, 1988.

López de Gómara, Francisco. *Cortés: the Life of the Conqueror by His Secretary*, trans. Lesley Byrd Simpson. Berkeley: University of California Press, 1964.

López Pinero, José Maria. "Las 'nuevas medicinas' americanas en la obra (1565–1574) de Nicolás Monardes." *Asclepio* 42(1990):3–68.

Lovejoy, Paul E., ed. *Africans in Bondage: Studies in Slavery and the Slave Trade*. Madison: University of Wisconsin Press, 1986.

Lovell, W. George. *Conquest and Survival in Colonial Guatemala: A Historical Geography of the Cuchumatán Highlands, 1500–1821*. Rev. ed. Montreal and Kingston: McGill-Queen's University Press, 1992.

Lovell, W. George. "Disease and Depopulation in Early Colonial Guatemala." In *The Secret Judgments of God: Native Peoples and Old World Disease in Colonial Spanish America*, ed. Noble David Cook and W. George Lovell, pp. 51–85. Norman: University of Oklahoma Press, 1992.

Lovell, W. George. "Enfermedades del Viejo Mundo y mortandad amerindia: La viruela y el tabardillo en la sierra de los Cuchumatanes de Guatemala (1780–1810)." *Mesoamerica* 16(1988):239–85.

Lovell, W. George. " 'Heavy Shadows and Black Night': Disease and Depopulation in Colonial Spanish America." *Annals of the Association of American Geographers* 82(1992):426–43.

McBryde, Felix Webster. "Influenza in America during the Sixteenth Century (Guatemala: 1523, 1559–1562, 1576)." *Bulletin of the History of Medicine* 8(1940):296–302.

McCaa, Robert. "Spanish and Nahuatl Views on Smallpox and Demographic Catastrophe in Mexico." *Journal of Interdisciplinary History* 25(1995):397–431.

MacCormack, Sabine. *Religion in the Andes. Vision and Imagination in Early Colonial Peru*. Princeton: Princeton University Press, 1991.

McCrady, Edward. *The History of South Carolina under the Proprietary Government, 1670–1719*. New York, 1897.

MacLeod, Murdo. *Spanish Central America: A Socioeconomic History, 1520–1720*. Berkeley: University of California Press, 1973.

McNeill, William H. *Plagues and Peoples*. Garden City, NY: Doubleday Anchor, 1976.

Major, R. H., ed. *Christopher Columbus: Four Voyages to the New World, Letters and Selected Documents*. Gloucester, MA: Peter Smith, 1978.

Malvido, Elsa. "Factores de despoblación y reposición de Cholula (1641–1810)." *Historia Mexicana* 89(1973):52–110.

Malvido, Elsa, and Carlos Viesca. "La epidémia de cocoliztli de 1576." *Historias* (México) 11(1985):27–33.

Manzano Manzano, Juan. *Los Pinzones y el descubrimiento de América*. 3 vols. Madrid, 1988.

Marks, G., and W. K. Beatty. *Epidemics*. New York: Scribner's, 1976.

Martin, Calvin. *The Keepers of the Game: Indian-Animal Relationships and the Fur Trade*. Berkeley: University of California Press, 1978.

Martínez Duran, Carlos. *Las ciencias médicas en Guatemala: origen y evolución*. Guatemala: Tipografía Sánchez y De Guise, 1941.

Mártir de Anglería, Pedro. *Décadas del Nuevo Mundo*. Buenos Aires: Editorial Bajel, 1944.

Matthias Lexers Mittelhochdeutsches Taschenwörterbuch. 36th ed. Leipzig: S. Hirzel Verlag, 1980.

Mendieta, Fray Jerónimo de. *Historia eclesiástica de México*. 4 vols. México: Editorial Salvador Chávez Hayhoe, 1945.

Menéndez Pidal, Ramón. *El padre Las Casas: Su doble personalidad*. Madrid: Espasa-Calpe, 1963.

Merbs, Charles F. "Patterns of Health and Sickness in the Precontact Southwest." *Precolumbian Consequences, Vol. I: Archaeological and Historical Perspectives on the Spanish Borderlands West*, ed. David Hurst Thomas, pp. 41–56. Washington, DC: Smithsonian Institution Press, 1989.

Mercer, A. J. "Smallpox and Epidemiological-Demographic Change in Europe: The Role of Vaccination." *Population Studies* 39(1985):287–307.

Milhou, A. *Colón y su mentalidad mesiánica en el ambiente franciscanista español*. Valladolid, 1983.

Miller, Joseph. "The Significance of Drought, Disease, and Famine in the Agriculturally Marginal Zones of West-Central Africa." *Journal of African History* 23(1982):17–61.

Millones, Luis, ed. *El retorno de las huacas: Estudios y documentos sobre el Taki Ongoy, Siglo XVI*. Lima: Instituto de Estudios Peruanos, 1990.

Milner, G. R. "Epidemic Disease in the Postcontact Southeast: A Reappraisal." *Midcontinental Journal of Archaeology* 5(1980):39–56.

Monardes, Nicolás. *Historia medicinal de las cosas que se traen de nuestras Indias occidentales que sirven en medicina* (1574, facs. ed.). Seville: Padilla Libros, 1988.

Morales Padrón, Francisco. *Andalucía y América*. Seville: Ediciones Guadalquivir, 1988.

Moreno Ollero, Antonio. *Sanlúcar de Barrameda a fines de la edad media.* Cádiz: Diputación Provincial de Cádiz, 1984.

Morison, Samuel Eliot. *Journals and Other Documents on the Life and Voyages of Christopher Columbus.* New York: Heritage Press, 1963.

Morison, Samuel Eliot. *The European Discovery of America. The Southern Voyages, 1492–1616.* New York: Oxford University Press, 1974.

Morton, Thomas. *New England Canaan.* Boston: Prince Society Publications, 1883.

Moseley, Michael E. *The Incas and Their Ancestors.* London: Thames & Hudson, 1992.

Motolinia o Benavente, Toribio de. *Memoriales o libro de las cosas de la Nueva España y de los naturales dello.* México: UNAM, 1971.

Moya Pons, Frank. *Después de Colón: Trabajo, sociedad y política en la economía del oro.* Madrid: Alianza Editorial, 1987.

Murra, John V. *The Economic Organization of the Inka State.* Greenwich, CT: JAI Press, 1980.

Newman, M. T. "Aboriginal New World Epidemiology and Medical Care, and the Impact of Old World Disease Imports." *American Journal of Physical Anthropology* 45(1976):667–72.

Newson, Linda A. *Indian Survival in Colonial Nicaragua.* Norman: University of Oklahoma Press, 1987.

Newson, Linda A. *Life and Death in Early Colonial Ecuador.* Norman: University of Oklahoma Press, 1995.

Newson, Linda A. "Old World Epidemics in Early Colonial Ecuador." In *The Secret Judgments of God: Native Peoples and Old World Disease in Colonial Spanish America,* ed. Noble David Cook and W. George Lovell, pp. 86–114. Norman: University of Oklahoma Press, 1992.

Newson, Linda A. *The Cost of Conquest: Indian Decline in Honduras under Spanish Rule.* Boulder, CO: Westview Press, 1986.

Newson, Linda A. "The Depopulation of Nicaragua in the Sixteenth Century." *Journal of Latin American Studies* 14(1982):253–86.

Numbers, Ronald L., ed. *Medicine in the New World: New Spain, New France, and New England.* Knoxville: University of Tennessee Press, 1987.

Núñez Cabeza de Vaca, Alvar. *Castaways. The Narrative of Alvar Núñez Cabeza de Vaca,* trans. Frances M. López-Morillas. Berkeley: University of California Press, 1993.

Oré, Luis Gerónimo de. *Relación histórica de la Florida, escrito en el siglo XVII.* 2 vols. Madrid, 1931–33.

Orellana, Sandra L. *Indian Medicine in Highland Guatemala.* Albuquerque: University of New Mexico Press, 1987.

Oviedo y Valdés, Gonzalo Fernández de. *Historia general y natural de las Indias, islas y Tierra Firme del mar océano.* 4 vols. Madrid: Imprenta de la Real Academia de Historia, 1851–55.

Oviedo y Valdés, Gonzalo Fernández de. *Sumario de la natural historia de las Indias*. México: Fondo de Cultura Económica, 1950.

Parkman, Francis. *The Conspiracy of Pontiac and the Indian War after the Conquest of Canada*. 9th ed., rev. Boston, 1883.

Parkman, Francis. *The Jesuits in North America in the Seventeenth Century*. Boston: New Library, 1909.

Parry, John H. "A Secular Sense of Responsibility." In *First Images of America: The Impact of the New World on the Old*, ed. Fredi Chiappelli. Berkeley: University of California Press, 1976.

Parry, John H. *The Age of Reconnaissance*. New York: World Publishing, 1963.

Patterson, K. David. "Bacillary Dysentery." In *The Cambridge World History of Human Disease*, ed. Kenneth F. Kiple, pp. 604–609. Cambridge: Cambridge University Press, 1993.

Patterson, K. David. *Pandemic Influenza, 1700–1900: A Study in Historical Epidemiology*. Totowa, NJ: Rowman & Littlefield, 1986.

Pease G. Y., Franklin, ed. *Collaguas I*. Lima: Pontificia Universidad Católica del Perú, 1977.

Pease G. Y., Franklin. *Los crónicas y los Andes*. Mexico City: Fondo de Cultura Económica, 1995.

Pérez Moreda, Vicente. *La crisis de mortalidad en la España interior (siglos XVI– XIX)*. Madrid: Siglo Veintiuno, 1980.

Phillips, William D., and Carla Rahn Phillips. *The Worlds of Christopher Columbus*. Cambridge: Cambridge University Press, 1992.

Pizarro, Pedro. *Relación del descubrimiento y conquista del Perú*. Lima: Pontificia Universidad Católica del Perú, 1978.

Pohl, Hans, ed. *The European Discovery of the World and Its Economic Effects on Pre-industrial Society, 1500–1800*. Stuttgart: Franz Steiner, 1990.

Polo, José Toribio. "Apuntes sobre las epidemias del Perú." *Revista Histórica* 5(1913):50–109.

Poma de Ayala, Felipe Guaman. *El primer nueva corónica y buen gobierno*, ed. John V. Murra and Rolena Adorno. 3 vols. México: Siglo Veintiuno, 1980.

Porras Barrenechea, Raúl, ed. *Cartas del Perú (1524–1543)*. Lima: Sociedad de Bibliófilos Peruanos, 1959.

Porras Barrenechea, Raúl. *Los cronistas del Perú (1528–1650) y otros ensayos*, ed. Franklin Pease G. Y. Lima: Banco de Crédito, 1986.

Powell, Mary Lucas. "Health and Disease in the Late Prehistoric Southeast." In *Disease and Demography in the Americas*, eds. John W. Verano and Douglas H. Ubelaker, pp. 41–53. Washington, DC: Smithsonian Institution Press, 1992.

Prem, Hanns J. "Disease Outbreaks in Central Mexico during the Sixteenth Century." In *The Secret Judgments of God: Native Peoples and Old World Disease in Colonial Spanish America*, ed. Noble David Cook and W. George Lovell, pp. 22–50. Norman: University of Oklahoma Press, 1992.

Purchas, Samuel. *Hakluytus Postumus; or, Purchas His Pilgrimes*. 20 vols. Glasgow: Maclehose, 1905–1907.

Quinn, David Beers, ed. *The Roanoke Voyages, 1584–1590*. 2 vols. London: Hakluyt Society, 1955.

Radell, David R. "The Indian Slave Trade and Population of Nicaragua during the Sixteenth Century." In *The Native Population of the Americas in 1492*, ed. Willian M. Denevan, pp. 67–76. 2nd ed. Madison: University of Wisconsin Press, 1992.

Ramenofsky, Ann F. *Vectors of Death: The Archaeology of European Contact*. Albuquerque: University of New Mexico Press, 1987.

Ravenholt, R. T. "Encephalitis Lethargica."In *The Cambridge World History of Human Disease*, ed. Kenneth F. Kiple, pp. 708–12. Cambridge: Cambridge University Press, 1993.

Recinos, Adrián, and Delia Goetz, eds. *The Annals of the Cakchiquels*. Norman: University of Oklahoma Press, 1953.

Reff, Daniel T. "Contact Shock in Northwestern New Spain, 1518–1764." In *Disease and Demography in the Americas*, ed. John W. Verano and Douglas H. Ubelaker, pp. 265–76. Washington, DC: Smithsonian Institution Press, 1992.

Reff, Daniel T. *Disease, Depopulation, and Culture Change in Northwestern New Spain, 1518–1764*. Salt Lake City: University of Utah Press, 1991.

Ricardo, Antonio. *Vocabulario y phrasis en la lengua general de los indios del Perú, llamada quichua*. Lima: San Marcos, 1951.

Rivera, Miguel, ed. *Chilam Balam de Chumayel*. Madrid: Historia 16, 1986.

Rodríguez Demorizi, Emilio. *Los dominicos y las encomiendas de indios de la isla Española*. Santo Domingo: Editora del Caribe, 1971.

Rosenblat, Angel. *La población de América en 1492: Viejos y nuevos cálculos*. México: Colegio de México, 1967.

Rosenblat, Angel. "The Population of Hispaniola at the Time of Columbus." In *The Native Population of the Americas in 1492*, 2nd ed., ed. William M. Denevan, pp. 43–66. Madison: University of Wisconsin Press, 1992.

Rostworowski de Diez Canseco, María. *Recursos naturales renovables y pesca, siglos XVI y XVII*. Lima: Instituto de Estudios Peruanos, 1981.

Rouse, Irving. *The Tainos, Rise and Decline of the People Who Greeted Columbus*. New Haven: Yale University Press, 1992.

Rutman, Darret B., and Anita H. Rutman. "Of Agues and Fevers: Malaria in the Early Chesapeake." *William and Mary Quarterly* 33 (1976):34–40.

Sahagún, Bernardino de. *Conquest of New Spain*. Salt Lake City: University of Utah Press, 1989.

Sahagún, Bernardino de. *Florentine Codex: General History of the Things of New Spain*, ed. Arthur J. O. Anderson and Charles E. Dibble. 13 in 12 vols. Santa Fe, NM: School of American Research, 1950–82.

Sahagún, Bernardino de. *Historia general de las cosas de Nueva España*, ed. Angel María Garibay K. México: Editorial Porrúa, 1992.

Sánchez-Albornoz, Nicolás. "Demographic Change in America and Africa Induced by the European Expansion, 1500–1800." In *The European Discovery of the World and Its Economic Effects on Pre-industrial Society, 1500–1800*, ed. Hans Pohl, pp. 195–206. Stuttgart: Franz Steiner, 1990.

Sánchez-Albornoz, Nicolás. *La población de América latina desde los tiempos precolombinos al año 2025*. Madrid: Alianza Editorial, 1994.

Sánchez-Albornoz, Nicolás, ed. *Población y mano de obra en América latina*. Madrid: Alianza Editorial, 1985.

Sánchez-Albornoz, Nicolás. *The Population of Latin America*. Berkeley: University of California Press, 1974.

Sánchez González, Ramón. "Hambres, pestes y guerras: Elementos de desequilibrio demográfico en la comarca de La Sagra durante la época moderna." *Hispania: Revista Española de Historia* 51 (1991):517–58.

Sandoval, Alonso de. *De Instaurando Aethiopum Salute* . . . Bogotá: Empresa Nacional de Publicaciones, 1956.

Santa Cruz Pachacuti Yamque, Juan. *Historia de los Incas*. Lima: Imprenta Sanmartí, 1927.

Sarmiento de Gamboa, Pedro. *Historia de los Incas*. Madrid: Ediciones Polifemo, 1988.

Sauer, Carl Ortwin. *The Early Spanish Main*. Berkeley: University of California Press, 1966.

Schafer, Ernesto. *El Consejo Real y Supremo de las Indias*. 2 vols. Seville: Centro de Estudios de Historia de América, 1935–1947.

Schmidel, Ulrich. *Relatos de la conquista del Rio de la Plata y Paraguay 1534–1554*. Madrid: Alianza Editorial, 1986.

Schwartz, S. B. *The Iberian Mediterranean and Atlantic Traditions in the Formation of Columbus as a Colonizer*. Minneapolis: University of Minnesota Press, 1986.

Sherman, William L. *Forced Native Labor in Sixteenth-Century Central America*. Lincoln: University of Nebraska Press, 1979.

Sinnecker, Herbert A. *General Epidemiology*. New York: Wiley, 1976.

Smith, Buckingham. *Relation of Alavar Núñez Cabeça de Vaca*. New York: J. Munsell, 1871.

Smith, Marvin T. *Archaeology of Aboriginal Culture Change in the Interior Southeast: Depopulation during the Early Historic Period*. Gainesville: University of Florida Press, 1987.

Soriano Lleras, Andrés. *La medicina en el Nuevo Reino de Granada durante la conquista y la colonia*. Bogotá, 1966.

Spalding, Karen. *Huarochirí: An Andean Society under Inca and Spanish Rule*. Stanford: Stanford University Press, 1984.

Stannard, David E. *American Holocaust. Columbus and the Conquest of the New World*. New York: Oxford University Press, 1992.

Stearn, Esther W., and Allen E. Stearn. *The Effect of Smallpox on the Destiny of the American Indian*. Boston, 1945.

Stern, Steve J. *Peru's Indian Peoples and the Challenge of Spanish Conquest: Huamanga to 1640*. Madison: University of Wisconsin Press, 1982.

Sticker, George. "Die Einschleppung europaischer Krankheiten in Amerika während der Entdeckunszeit; ihr Einfluss auf den Rückgang der Bevölkerung." *Ibero-Amerikanisches Archiv* 6 (1932–33):62–83, 194–224.

Stodder, Ann L. W., and Debra L. Martin. "Health and Disease in the Southwest before and after Spanish Contact." In *Disease and Demography in the Americas*, ed. John W. Verano and Douglas H. Ubelaker, pp. 55–73. Washington, DC: Smithsonian Institution Press, 1992.

Suardo, Juan Antonio. *Diario de Lima (1629–1634)*. Lima: Vásquez, 1935.

Swanton, John R. *Indians of the Southeastern United States*. Bulletin 137. Washington, DC: Bureau of American Ethnology, 1946.

Sweet, David G. "The Population of the Upper Amazon Valley, Seventeenth and Eighteenth Centuries." M.A. thesis. Madison: University of Wisconsin, 1969.

Thevet, André. *La Cosmographie universelle*. Paris, 1575.

Thomas, David Hurst, ed. *Columbian Consequences, vol. I. Archaeological and Historical Perspectives on the Spanish Borderlands West*. 2 vols. Washington, DC: Smithsonian Institution Press, 1989.

Thornton, Russell. *American Indian Holocaust and Survival: A Population History since 1492*. Norman: University of Oklahoma Press, 1987.

Tio, Aurelio. *Dr. Diego Alvarez Chanca: Estudio biográfico*. San Germán, PR, 1966.

Torquemada, Juan de. *Monarquía indiana*. Madrid: Rodríguez Franco, 1723.

Torre, Tomás de la. *Diario de viaje de Salamanca a Chiapa, 1544–1545*. Caleruega, Burgos: Editorial OPE, 1985.

Torres de Mendoza, L., ed. *Colección de documentos inéditos relativos al descubrimiento, conquista y colonización de las posesiones españolas en América y Oceanía*. 42 vols. Madrid, 1864–1884.

Traboulay, David M. *Columbus and Las Casas: The Conquest and Christianization of America, 1492–1566*. New York: University Press of America, 1995.

Varner, John Grier, and Jeannette Johnson Varner, trans. and eds. *The Florida of the Inca by Garcilaso de la Vega*. Austin: University of Texas Press, 1988.

Vaughan, Alden T. *New England Frontier: Puritans and Indians 1620–1675*. Boston: Little, Brown, 1965.

Vázquez, Francisco. *Crónica de la provincia del santísimo nombre de Jesús de Guatemala*. Guatemala: Sociedad de Geografía e Historia, 1937.

Vázquez de Ayllón, Lucas. "Relación que hizo el licenciado Lucas Vázquez de Ayllón, de sus diligencias para estorbar el rompimiento entre Cortés y

Narváez." In *Cartas y relaciones de Hernán Cortés al Emperador Carlos V*, ed. Pascual de Gayangos. Paris, 1866.

Verano, John W. "Prehistoric Disease and Demography in the Andes." In *Disease and Demography in the Americas*, ed. John W. Verano and Douglas H. Ubelaker, pp. 15–24. Washington, DC: Smithsonian Institution Press, 1992.

Verano, John W., and Douglas H. Ubelaker, eds. *Disease and Demography in the Americas*. Washington, DC: Smithsonian Institution Press, 1992.

Verlinden, Charles. "La population de l'Amérique précolumbienne: Une question de méthode." In *Méthodologie de l'histoire et des sciences humaines: mélanges en honneur de Fernand Braudel*, pp. 453–62. Paris, 1973.

Villamarin, Juan A., and Judith E. Villamarin. "Epidemic Disease in the Sabana de Bogotá, 1536–1810." In *The Secret Judgments of God: Native Peoples and Old World Disease in Colonial Spanish America*, ed. Noble David Cook and W. George Lovell, pp. 115–43. Norman: University of Oklahoma Press, 1992.

Vincent, Bernard. "Las epidemias en Andalucía durante el siglo XVI." *Asclepio* 29 (1977):351–58.

Walter, John, and Roger Schofield, eds. *Famine, Disease and the Social Order in Early Modern Society*. Cambridge: Cambridge University Press, 1989.

Watts, David. *The West Indies: Patterns of Development, Culture and Environmental Change since 1492*. Cambridge: Cambridge University Press, 1987.

Way, A. B. "Diseases of Latin America." In *Biocultural Aspects of Disease*, ed. H. Rothschild, pp. 253–91. New York: Academic Press, 1981.

Weissmann, Gerald. "They All Laughed at Christopher Columbus." *Hospital Practice* 21 (15 January 1986):30–37, 41.

Whitmore, Thomas M. *Disease and Death in Early Colonial Mexico. Simulating Amerindian Depopulation*. Boulder, CO: Westview Press, 1992.

Williams, Herbert U. "Epidemics among Indians, 1616–1620." *Johns Hopkins Hospital Bulletin* 20 (1909):340–49.

Wilson, Samuel L. *Hispaniola: Caribbean Chiefdoms in the Age of Columbus*. Tuscaloosa: University of Alabama Press, 1990.

Winthrop, John. *Winthrop Papers, 1631–1637*. Boston: Massachusetts Historical Society, 1943.

Winthrop, Robert C. *Life and Letters of John Winthrop*. 2 vols. Boston: Ticknor & Fields, 1864–67.

Wood, Peter H. "The Impact of Smallpox on the Native Population of the Eighteenth Century South." *New York State Journal of Medicine* 87 (1987):30.

Wood, William. *New England's Prospect* [1634]. Amherst: University of Massachusetts Press, 1977.

Wright, Ronald. *Stolen Continents: The Americas through Indian Eyes since 1492*. New York: Houghton Mifflin, 1992.

Zambardino, Rudolph A. "Critique of David Henige's 'On the Contact Population of Hispaniola: History as Higher Mathematics.' " *Hispanic American Historical Review* 58 (1978):700–708.

Zambardino, Rudolph A. "Mexico's Population in the Sixteenth Century: Demographic Anomaly or Mathematical Illusion?" *Journal of Interdisciplinary History* 11 (1980):1–27.

Zavala, Silvio. *El servicio personal de los indios en el Perú*. 3 vols. México: El Colegio de México, 1978–80.

Zavala, Silvio. *La encomienda indiana*. 2nd ed. México: Editorial Porrúa, 1975.

Ziegler, Philip. *The Black Death*. Hammondsworth: Pelican Books, 1976.

Zinnser, Hans. *Rats, Lice and History*. New York: Bantam Books, 1960.

INDEX